Walther H. W. Schulze

ECG Imaging of Ventricular Activity in Clinical Applications

Vol. 22
Karlsruhe Transactions on Biomedical Engineering

Editor:
Karlsruhe Institute of Technology (KIT)
Institute of Biomedical Engineering

Eine Übersicht aller bisher in dieser Schriftenreihe erschienenen Bände finden Sie am Ende des Buchs.

ECG Imaging of Ventricular Activity in Clinical Applications

by
Walther H. W. Schulze

KIT Scientific Publishing

Dissertation, Karlsruher Institut für Technologie (KIT)
Fakultät für Elektrotechnik und Informationstechnik, 2015
Referenten: Prof. Dr. rer. nat. Olaf Dössel
Prof. Dr.-Ing. habil. Jens Haueisen

Impressum

KIT Scientific Publishing

Karlsruher Institut für Technologie (KIT)
KIT Scientific Publishing
Straße am Forum 2
D-76131 Karlsruhe

www.ksp.kit.edu

Print on Demand 2015

ISSN 1864-5933
ISBN 978-3-7315-0374-3
DOI 10.5445/KSP/1000046918

ECG Imaging of Ventricular Activity in Clinical Applications

Zur Erlangung des akademischen Grades eines

DOKTOR-INGENIEURS

von der Fakultät für

Elektrotechnik und Informationstechnik

des Karlsruher Instituts für Technologie (KIT)

genehmigte

DISSERTATION

von

Dipl.-Ing. Walther Hermann Wolfgang Schulze

geb. in Gifhorn

Tag der mündlichen Prüfung:	16. Februar 2015
Hauptreferent:	Prof. Dr. rer. nat. Olaf Dössel
Korreferent:	Prof. Dr.-Ing. habil. Jens Haueisen

Contents

Part IV Discussion

Part V Appendix

Acknowledgements

Although it may be broadly accepted that progress is driven by imagination, the benefit of research for society is usually uncertain and its effects take often quite indirect paths. Hence, I am grateful to those who gave hard-earned resources to make this work possible:

Initially, in the first months, the European Community with its Seventh Framework Programme (FP7/2007-2013) under grant agreement no 224495 (euHeart project), the German Research Foundation under grants DO637/10-1 and DO637/13-1, the Karlsruhe House of Young Scientists (KHYS) Networking Grant and finally a scholarship by the Graduate Funding from the German States.

This thesis was conducted under supervision of Olaf Dössel at the Institute of Biomedical Engineering, Karlsruhe Institute of Technology (KIT). I would like to thank him and Prof. Dr.-Ing. habil. Jens Haueisen sincerely for their efforts in reviewing this work and for making the defense of this thesis possible.
At the institute, I was received into a fruitful and indeed perfect environment, with great organizational infrastructure and perfect financial support for the conducted research, and most importantly with amazing people. The open, cooperative culture, the sharing of ideas, distributed responsibilities and the inspiration and drive towards reaching scientific goals were essential to make this work evolve.
I would like to express my deepest thanks for being part of this team. Among those who contributed directly to this work, I would like to thank Danila Potyagaylo for introducing me to the best of Russian ska music, Yuan Jiang for negotiating and drafting research proposals while

in Wuhan, Martin Krüger for rocking the euHeart project, Thomas Fritz for his restless efforts in producing personalized jokes and smart hacks of any kind, Axel Loewe for his elaborate sense of good taste, culture and manners, Goofy for keeping up that enthusiastic spirit, David Keller for betting his property on my sprinting talents and Mathias Wilhelms and Frank Weber for proving that good things should be short and to the point. I would like to thank Mrs. Günter for the excellent cooperation and Manfred Schroll for keeping our flow of bits and bytes alive. Finally, I would like to thank Olaf Dössel for being constantly available to the entire group, for his unparalleled commitment and enthusiasm, his confidence in individual responsibility that made many initiatives possible and for forming this team together with Gunnar Seemann over years.

Further, I would like to thank my students for their excellent contributions to this work: Biao Wang, Alexander von Lühmann, Francesc Elies Henar, Dan-Timon Rudolph, Patrick Mackens, Kathryn Vogel, Rasmus Jones, Eulàlia Mascareñas Marsal, Esraa Ragaa Khaled Fattoh, Christian Ritter, Vynnie Kong, Julia Trächtler, and further Eike Wülfers and Mrs. Schyma for their support.

Further, for being great colleagues, Oussama Jarrousse, Matthias Keller, Tobias Baas, Tobias Oesterlein, Bhawna Verma, Jochen Schmidt, Lukas Baron, Stefan Pollnow, Markus Rottmann, Christopher Schilling, Julia Bohnert, Sebastian Seitz, Ramona Modery, Charis Kahlmeyer and Dirk Falkenberg.

At University Medical Center Mannheim, the clinical PVC study for this thesis has grown in an excellent and trustful cooperation under the lead of Prof. Dr. med. Rainer Schimpf. I would like to express my thanks to the entire team of clinical researchers involved in the study, namely Prof. Dr. med. Theano Papavassiliu, Dr. med. Erol Tülümen, Dr. med. Boris Rudic, Dr. med. Volker Liebe, PD Dr. med. Christina Dösch, PD Dr. med. Torsten Konrad, Dr. med. Christian Veltmann and Prof. Dr. med. Martin Borggrefe.

For conducting the VT study, I would like to thank Dr. Kawal Rhode and Dr. Zhong Chen as well as Professor Aldo Rinaldi and Professor Reza Razavi of King's College London, and further Dr. Jatin Relan and Dr. Hervé Delingette of INRIA, Sophia Antipolis.

Finally, I would like to thank Andreas Bierfreund for his enthusiasm in teaching maths and physics, the SZ Jägercorps Knesebeck e.V. for being the best band in the world, the Konrad-Adenauer-Stiftung for their support of my studies and my parents and my sister for their support, encouragement, belief and care along the entire way.

1 Introduction

This chapter will give an impression on why it is fascinating to solve the inverse problem of ECG. Further, an abstract is written for the busy reader.

The fascination of solving the inverse problem of electrocardiography

Cardiac mechanical activity is triggered by a wavefront-like electric excitation spread between the cells of the myocardium. In this work, the goal is to visualize such electric activity using electric field calculation and measurements of ECG signals on the body surface (body surface potential maps).

ECG signals on the body surface are the smoothed out result of the electric signals in the heart. When reverse-computing the sources from a measured ECG, the damping of the body must be inverted, which leads to strong amplification of any noise in the ECG or the model. In addition, the solution of the inverse problem of ECG is not unique. Multiple combinations of sources may result in the same ECG.

Hence, ECG imaging provides a broad playground for mathematical methods that reaches from making realistic patient models to solving the *ill-posed* inverse problem. For the latter, this includes regularization, optimization and signal processing. The goal is to introduce generic physiological knowledge on the sought inverse solution in order to stabilize the solution and cope with its ambiguity — without introducing information that is sought for or artifacts that could lead to false conclusions. On top of that, all these methods are applied in a clinical environment, which includes patients and challenges such as usability, robustness and reliability.

Abstract

The goal of this research is to visualize electrical activity in the cardiac muscle solely from non-invasive measurements, i.e. from a multichannel electrocardiogram (body surface potential map, BSPM) combined with computer models of the human thorax and heart which are built from MRI-scans. In particular and in contrast to most existing works, cardiac electric activity is reconstructed across the myocardial wall — either as transmembrane voltages (TMVs) over time or as activation times — and a validation study of the method is performed in patients with premature ventricular contractions (PVCs) and ventricular tachycardia (VT). In the validation study, existing algorithms have been tested on volumetric models and surface models (endo- and epicardium), and a few new approaches for ECG imaging of TMVs and activation times have been developed.

Structure

This work presents results of

- a clinical validation study that presents the ability of ECG imaging of localizing ventricular excitation origins and of imaging activation times of related beats (see Sect. 7.1) and secondly,
- a clinical validation study that presents the ability of ECG imaging of imaging activation times of sustained monomorphic ventricular tachycardia (see Sect. 7.2).

Further, in terms of methods, it presents

- a processing framework for the clinical validation studies (see Sect. 6)
- a camera system that allows for instantaneous and automatic localization of BSPM electrodes in the catheter lab (see Sect. 6.2)
- new ECG imaging approaches that introduce knowledge from a dynamic model of the cardiac excitation propagation (see Sect.5.1)

- a framework to enhance ECG imaging solutions with single intracardiac measurements during ablation procedures with little arrhythmic activity (see Sect. 5.3)
- a spatio-temporal Tikhonov method that identifies the optimal offset in the BSPM (see Sect. 5.4)
- a BSPM smoother that identifies the optimal BSPM offset through optimization of its smoothness and by minimization of its energy (see Eq. 6.10)
- a new variant of the critical times method (see Sect. 5.2)
- a simple model-based ECG imaging approach that performed best among the methods for FEM-models (see Sect. 5.5)

Abbreviations

ATintT2 - activation time imaging, time integral, Sect. 4.3.4
BEM - boundary element method
BSPM - body surface potential map
CritTeff35 - critical times method, Sect. 4.3.5
ECG - electrocardiogram
ECGI - electrocardiographic imaging
EFF - effective pacing
EPU - electrophysiological unit
FEM - finite element method
KCL - King's College London
LAT - local activation time
LV/RV - left/right ventricle
LVOT/RVOT - left/right ventricular outflow tract
MAP - maximum a posteriori method, Sect. 4.3.3
MAPSTwin, MAPSTqrs - spatio-temporal variants of MAP
MODcct, MODccs - model-based approaches, Sect. 5.5
OFF, OFFR - spatio-temporal method with offset correction, Sect. 5.4
PVC - premature ventricular contraction
R-20 - BSPM signal at 20% of the QRS length before the R-peak
STD - standard deviation
Tikh - Tikhonov regularization, Sect. 4.3.1
TikhGS - Tikhonov-Greensite regularization, Sect. 4.3.2
TMV - transmembrane voltage
UMM - University Medical Center Mannheim
VT - ventricular tachycardia

Part I

Fundamentals

2

Medical Motivation and Fundamentals

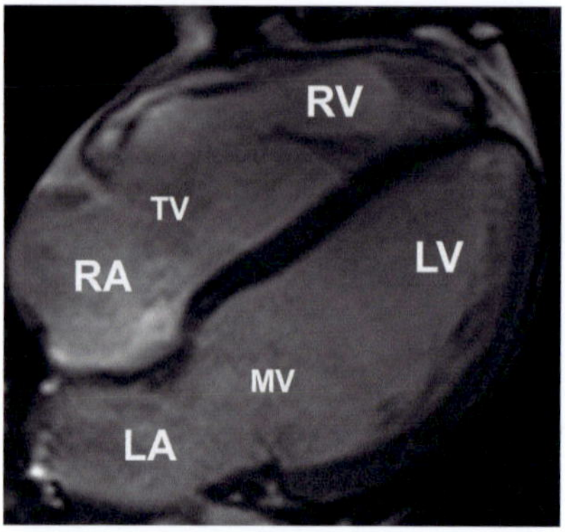

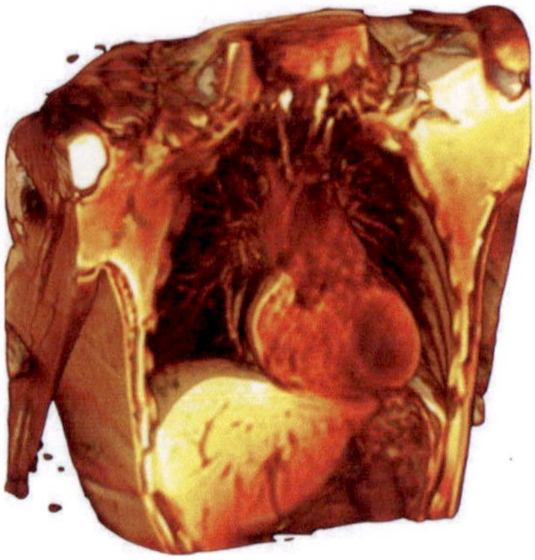

Figure 2.1: The heart as seen in cardiac cine MRI (left) and in context of the thorax (right, MRI, volumetric interpolated breath-hold examination). Patient 15, M, healthy. LV/RV: left/right ventricle, LA/RA: left/right atrium, MV/TV: mitral/tricuspid valve.

The heart is a muscular organ, and its proper functioning is of vital nature. The mechanical behaviour of the heart is controlled by electric excitation in the myocardial tissue that triggers the release of calcium and thereby the contraction of the muscle fibers (an MR image of cardiac muscle is depicted in Fig. 2.1 (left) for the atria and ventricles). In the case of cardiac arrhythmia, the patterns of electric excitation conduction are pathological, which causes a reduced efficiency of its pumping mechanism, leading to reduced blood supply to the pulmonary and systemic circulation systems, which are partially visible along with the heart in the thorax MRI scan of Fig. 2.1 (right).
Hence, to diagnose cardiac arrhythmia, the cardiac electric activity has to be studied, which is typically done non-invasively by the 12-lead ECG — and then confirmed with catheter measurements during ablation therapies, which are performed in catheter laboratories or electrophysiological units (EPUs). In such therapies, cardiac substrates are ablated to change the pathways of electric excitation conduction. Such therapies are often stressful for the patient, logistically expensive, and they usually take several hours, with low success rates, e.g. in case of atrial fibrillation. This work shall improve the accuracy of non-invasive pre-interventional diagnosis and shall facilitate better

treatment planning of such therapies. It also suggests a method to produce electroanatomical maps from fewer measurements, which is important in the case of sparse arrhythmic activity that often leads to termination of long-planned catheter lab studies.
The central validation study of this thesis deals with ECG imaging of premature ventricular contractions (PVCs). To treat this kind of arrhythmia, which has an ectopic, focal excitation origin, protocols such as the following three-phase mapping procedure are typically a guide for cardiologists. While most cardiologists decide based on personal experience rather than computed results, the following scheme represents a computer-aided algorithm of finding the focus of the excitation. The algorithm is used here to reflect the state-of-the art for methods that do not take advantage of anatomical models from MRI or CT, which are used in ECG imaging.

Three-phase mapping procedure: pace mapping and treatment of PVCs

To localize the foci of ectopic beats and the excitation paths of cardiac arrhythmia in general, patients are usually subjected to invasive catheter pacing studies. A catheter is placed in the endocardium and pacings are performed to imitate the sought beat. Patterns of the electrocardiograms found beforehand for PVCs are then compared with the ECGs that result from the pacing - a procedure called pace mapping. Pace mappings can be performed heuristically or according to formalistic protocols. In a systematic approach by Peeters et al. [1], pace mapping is performed using the following three-phase strategy [2]:

- The QRS integral of the sought arrhythmia is computed for the channels of a BSPM. A database of QRS integral maps is then created, using the mean QRS integral found for pacings at a certain pacing location. The initial estimate for the target location is then selected from the database using the correlation coefficient between the database signal and the sought signal.
- In the area of the target location, new pacings are then performed, and their QRS integral is again compared with that of the sought arrhythmia and other paced signals in the area that are already in

the database, until a good match is found. During the procedure the catheter is guided using biplane X-ray imaging.

- Finally, local activation sequence mapping is performed for the PVCs to find the site of earliest activation. This site is then used to perform the radiofrequency ablation therapy.

Medical Motivation

The medical motivation of this work is to make computer models of the volume conductor of the human body available for improved treatment planning that does not rely on pace mapping, but computes visualizations of the cardiac electric activity based on information from field calculations. The goal is to improve the quality of estimates of the excitation origin, to reduce the time and stress of ablation procedures and the number of required pacings, and to avoid termination of procedures in case of sparse arrhythmic activity (for an overview of the procedure durations in this study, see Tab. B.2 on page 167).

3

Mathematical and Biophysical Fundamentals

This chapter introduces the underlying principles of forward calculations that are used in computer models of the heart. It gives an overview of the Maxwell equations and introduces the basic foundations of the forward calculations (a comprehensive introduction is given in the books by Gulrajani [3] and Malmivuo [4]). Also, a basic introduction to signal processing is given to specify what filters have been used to deal with measured signals of BSPMs in this work. Fundamentals of the inverse problem of ECG are given in Sect. 4.

3.1 Maxwell's Equations and Bioelectric Fields

To understand bioelectric or biomagnetic fields, a good understanding of the behaviour and interaction of the respective fields and their sources is required. These are typically framed by the following set of equations, which is named after James Clerk Maxwell, in honour of his publications in the field in 1861 [5] and thereafter.

Gauss's Law

The charge is the source of the electric field [3, Chapt. 5.2][6]:

$$\nabla \cdot \vec{D} = \rho \tag{3.1}$$

$$\Leftrightarrow \oiint_{\partial V} \vec{D} \cdot \mathrm{d}\vec{a} = \iiint_V \nabla \cdot \vec{D} \mathrm{d}v = \iiint_V \rho \mathrm{d}v = Q, \tag{3.2}$$

$$\vec{E} = \frac{\vec{D} - \vec{P}}{\varepsilon_0} \tag{3.3}$$

Where $\vec{E}$ is the electric field and $\vec{D}$ the electric displacement field, ρ the free charge density and Q the free charge. ρ results in $\vec{D}$.

Gauss's Law for Magnetism

There are no point sources or point sinks [1] in magnetic fields [3, Chapt. 5.2][6]:

$$\nabla \cdot \vec{B} = 0 \tag{3.4}$$

$$\Leftrightarrow \oint\!\!\!\oint_{\partial V} \vec{B} \cdot \mathrm{d}\vec{a} = 0, \tag{3.5}$$

$$\vec{H} = \frac{\vec{B}}{\mu_0} - \vec{M} \tag{3.6}$$

Maxwell's equations are presented in their macroscopic form here, which focuses on the free charges and free currents. Equations 3.3 and 3.6 are called the material equations, where ε_0 and μ_0 are the vacuum permittivity and permeability [3, Chapt. 5.2]. While in vacuum, there is only an electric field of free charges, the electric field $\vec{E}$ in a material represents also the polarization $\vec{P}$ of the atoms and bound electrons. For this reason, $\vec{D}$ is introduced as the field that is created solely by free charges. Analogously, the magnetic field $\vec{H}$ is composed of the magnetic flux density $\vec{B}$ and the magnetization $\vec{M}$ of the material.
With a similar equation, the resulting current density through a medium can be described as the composition of a field-induced conduction current density $\sigma\vec{E}$ and an impressed current density $\vec{J^i}$ [3, Chapt. 5.2]:

$$\vec{J} = \sigma\vec{E} + \vec{J^i} \tag{3.7}$$

As $\vec{P}$ is created by pairs of bounded positive and negative charges of equal size and opposite sign and $\vec{M}$ is created by bounded pairs of north- and southpoles, the impressed currents $\vec{J^i}$ are created by pairs of current sources of equal size and opposite sign.

[1] Note that recent research has shown experimental hints for the existence of magnetic monopoles under specific conditions [7, 8].

Faraday's Law of Induction

For the non-stationary case and for magnetic fields, another two laws apply. First, a changing magnetic field causes a curl in the electric field [3, Chapt. 5.2]:

$$\nabla \times \vec{E} = -\frac{\partial \vec{B}}{\partial t}, \tag{3.8}$$

or with Stokes' theorem and an open surface S:

$$\Leftrightarrow \iint_S (\nabla \times \vec{E}) \cdot \mathrm{d}\vec{a} = \oint_{\partial S} \vec{E} \cdot \mathrm{d}\vec{l} = -\iint_S \frac{\partial \vec{B}}{\partial t} \cdot \mathrm{d}\vec{a} := -\frac{\partial \Phi_B}{\partial t}, \tag{3.9}$$

where Φ_B is called the magnetic flux (unit: Tm^2).

Ampère's Circuital Law

On the other hand, a changing electric displacement field and a free current density cause a curl in the magnetic field [3, Chapt. 5.2]:

$$\nabla \times \vec{H} = \vec{J} + \frac{\partial \vec{D}}{\partial t} \tag{3.10}$$

From these equations it was possible to predict the dynamic coupling of electric and magnetic fields and from that the existence of electromagnetic waves. This hypothesis was confirmed by Heinrich Hertz in 1887 [6].

3.2 Forward Calculation of Bioelectric Fields

Quasi-Static Approximation

For the electric and magnetic fields that are produced by the human heart and body, the temporal derivatives in Faraday's law and Ampère's law can be neglected [9] (for a detailed explanation, see [3, Chapt. 5.3]), i.e.

$$\nabla \times \vec{E} \approx 0 \tag{3.11}$$

$$\nabla \times \vec{H} \approx \vec{J}. \tag{3.12}$$

Bidomain Model

The bidomain (or bisyncytial) model [10] that is used to calculate bioelectric and biomagnetic fields makes use of this approximation. Since the divergence of the curl is zero, the following relationship can be derived from Eq. 3.10, given the approximation in Eq. 3.12:

$$\nabla \cdot (\nabla \times \vec{H}) = \nabla \cdot \vec{J} = 0. \tag{3.13}$$

With $\vec{E} = -\nabla\varphi$ and Eq. 3.7 this yields

$$\nabla \cdot (\sigma \vec{E} + \vec{J^i}) = 0 \tag{3.14}$$

$$\Leftrightarrow \nabla \cdot (\sigma \nabla \varphi) = \nabla \cdot \vec{J^i}, \tag{3.15}$$

where $\nabla \cdot \vec{J^i} = -I_{sv}$ represents impressed currents as a volume current source density in A/m^3, which is defined positive $I_{sv} > 0$ for when an impressed current goes into the volume conductor [11, Sect. 3.2.2].
For the active myocardium, impressed currents originate at the cell membranes. To model the complex structure of cardiac cells and tissue fibers that may cause these impressed currents, a second domain was introduced by [10], which represents intra- and extracellular space as a bidomain model, in which the two domains coexist in space. Current densities in the intra-cellular domain are now modeled as $\vec{J}_i = \sigma_i \vec{E}_i$ and those in the extra-cellular space as $\vec{J}_e = \sigma_e \vec{E}_e$, producing a current density of $\vec{J} = \vec{J}_i + \vec{J}_e$. The two domains are linked through the cell membrane. With Eq. 3.13, the following continuity equation must hold:

$$\nabla \cdot (\vec{J_i} + \vec{J_e}) = 0 \tag{3.16}$$

$$\Leftrightarrow \nabla \cdot (\sigma_i \nabla \varphi_i + \sigma_e \nabla \varphi_e) = 0, \tag{3.17}$$

where σ_i and σ_e need to be modeled as tensors due to the anisotropic nature of the conductivities in the heart. Defining the transmembrane voltage (TMV) as $V_m = \varphi_i - \varphi_e$, this yields

$$\nabla \cdot ((\sigma_i + \sigma_e) \nabla \varphi_e + \sigma_i \nabla V_m) = 0 \tag{3.18}$$

$$\Leftrightarrow \nabla \cdot ((\sigma_i + \sigma_e) \nabla \varphi_e) = -\nabla \cdot (\sigma_i \nabla V_m) = -I_{sv}, \tag{3.19}$$

which for $\sigma = \sigma_i + \sigma_e$ yields a Poisson's equation similar to Eq. 3.15. The equation can be solved for the entire volume conductor when adjusting σ locally ($\sigma_i = 0$ for the region outside the active myocardium) and introducing on the right-hand-side an impressed current source density $-I_{sv}$ that originates, e.g. from the setting of V_m in the calculation of the lead field matrix.
This Poisson's problem can be solved with the finite element method as explained in [11], using the following boundary conditions at the discontinuities of the conductivities, where φ_t denotes φ_e in the volume conductor outside the myocardium [12, 13]:

$$\varphi_e = \varphi_t \quad \text{at the heart surface} \tag{3.20}$$
$$\sigma_e \nabla \varphi_e \cdot \vec{n} = \sigma_t \nabla \varphi_t \cdot \vec{n} \quad \text{at the heart surface} \tag{3.21}$$
$$\sigma_i \nabla \varphi_i \cdot \vec{n} = 0 \quad \text{at the heart surface} \tag{3.22}$$
$$\sigma_t \nabla \varphi_t \cdot \vec{n} = 0 \quad \text{at the thorax surface} \tag{3.23}$$
$$\varphi_t = 0 \quad \text{at the point of the ground electrode} \tag{3.24}$$

In that order, these conditions are imposed for continuity to hold on the boundary between the heart and thorax tissues, for the conservation of charge that goes as current densities from the extracellular domain of the heart into the domain of the extracellular potentials in the thorax, further to not allow the intracellular currents to leave their domain at the heart surface, and for the extracellular currents in the thorax not to leave the body. Finally, for the solution to be unique, the point of the BSPM ground electrode is set to 0.

Boundary Element Method

For the boundary element method, conductivites in Eq. 3.19 are assumed to be isotropic. Given isotropic conductivity of the myocardium, only the TMVs at the surface of the heart produce a source of the BSPM [14]. The Poisson's problem of Eq. 3.19 can then be solved as a surface integral that is represented by the $k = 2$ surfaces of the thorax and heart (endo- and epicardium), each of which are conductivity interfaces with homogeneous conductivities specified for their inner and outer sides. This results in two pairs: the conductivities of the heart and thorax, and those of the thorax and air. In addition, an intracellular effective conductivity is specified for the heart [15]. The TMV distribution at the cardiac surface is then introduced as the source in [15, Eq.1], which is solved after the body surface potentials with the Matlab toolbox provided in [16].

3.3 Signal Processing

This section provides fundamentals for the very basic filtering methods used in this work.

Inner Product The inner product of two energy signals is defined as [17, Eq. 3.10]:

$$\langle x(t), y(t)\rangle = \int_{-\infty}^{\infty} x(t)y(t)dt,\ x(t)\in\mathbb{R},\ y(t)\in\mathbb{R} \tag{3.25}$$

The inner product is represented in the correlation function $r_{xy}(\tau)$ at $\tau = 0$.

Convolution The convolution of two signals is defined as the following inner product [17, Eq. 3.135]:

$$h(t)*y(t) = \langle h(t-\tau), y(\tau)\rangle_\tau = \int_{-\infty}^{\infty} h(t-\tau)y(\tau)d\tau. \tag{3.26}$$

It can be shown that

$$y(t)*h(t) = y(t)*h(t),\ \ y(t)*\delta(t) = y(t). \tag{3.27}$$

Fourier transform The Fourier transform computes the convolution of $y(t)$ with harmonic functions of a given frequency. As the convolution is performed with a co-sinus in the real and a sinus, which is a co-sinus shifted in time, in the complex domain ($e^{-j2\pi ft} = cos(2\pi ft) - jsin(2\pi ft)$), the resulting Fourier transform is a complex number that represents both the amplitude and time shift for a given frequency f [17, Eq. 3.124].

$$\mathscr{F}\{y(t)\} = Y(f) = \int_{-\infty}^{\infty} y(t) e^{-j2\pi f t} dt \tag{3.28}$$

Filtering Linear time-invariant filters are characterized by their impulse response function $h(t)$ or its Fourier transform $H(f)$, the transfer function. Convolving a signal with $h(t)$ is equivalent to multiplying it with $H(f)$ in frequency domain:

$$\begin{aligned} y(t) &= x(t) * h(t) \\ \mathscr{F}\{y(t)\} &= Y(f) = X(f)H(f) \end{aligned} \tag{3.29}$$

Gaussian High-Pass and Low-Pass Filters Low pass and high pass filters can be designed using the Gaussian bell in frequency space as transfer function, for low-pass:

$$H(f) = e^{\frac{-f^2}{2\sigma_f^2}} \tag{3.30}$$

or for high-pass filter characteristics ($H(f) = 1$ would yield an all-pass filter, subtracting a Gaussian bell leads to a stop band in $H(f)$):

$$H(f) = 1 - e^{\frac{-f^2}{2\sigma_f^2}}. \tag{3.31}$$

The tuning parameter of the Gaussian filter is the standard deviation of the Gaussian bell σ_f. $H(f)$ is typically assumed to have an effect of $-3\,\text{dB}$ (corresponding to a gain of $1/\sqrt{2}$) for the desired cutoff frequency f_c or an effect of $1/2$ on the power spectrum. In this work, for the Gaussian filter design, however, f_c is defined as the $-6\,\text{dB}$ cutoff frequency, with an effect of $1/2$ on the signal amplitude [18]:

$$H(f_c) = e^{\frac{-f_c^2}{2\sigma_f^2}} = \frac{1}{2} \tag{3.32}$$

$$\Leftarrow \sigma_f = \frac{f_c}{\sqrt{2ln(2)}} \tag{3.33}$$

Notch Filter A stop band filter produces a stop band in the frequency domain, i.e., a certain range of frequencies does not pass the filter. For a notch filter, stop bands are very narrow ("notc'h"). They may be applied periodically in frequency domain in order to eliminate a specific frequency f_n and its harmonics, e.g. power line hum. A Gaussian-based notch filter may therefore be designed using the following transfer function:

$$H(f) = 1 - \sum_{k=1}^{N} e^{-\frac{-(f-f_n k)^2}{2\sigma_f^2}}, \tag{3.34}$$

$$N = \left\lfloor \frac{f_s}{2f_n} \right\rfloor \tag{3.35}$$

where Gaussian filters of "standard deviation" σ_f are used. Periodic repetitions of the Gaussian notches are needed up to a shift by the Nyquist frequency, which is half the sampling frequency. This is due to discrete signals being represented only up to the Nyquist frequency in digital computers, as the highest frequency in a sampled signal is that over any two samples in time.

Part II

Methods

4

The State-of-the-Art in ECG Imaging

"The upcoming years will be crucial for ECG imaging, as it is getting a lot of attention through commercialization. It will have this chance once, and either it will be accepted, or it will fail to convince physicians and people will not touch it for a long time."

Rob MacLeod

This chapter will give an introduction to the inverse problem of ECG, its ill-posedness and to typical solvers of the problem that have been used in this work for the clinical studies, Sect. 7. It will then give an overview of the state-of-the-art in the field, with a focus on clinical validation studies. Finally, an outline is given on modeling errors that need to be tackled to facilitate a proper quality of results in the case of clinical data.

4.1 Linear Formulation of the Forward Problem of ECG

To solve the inverse problem of ECG, which is to compute cardiac electric sources from body surface potential maps, a model of the forward problem is required. In this work, this was primarily based on calculations with the finite element method (FEM) [11, 19] and the bidomain model in Sect. 3.2. Alternatively, the boundary element method (BEM) [15, 16, 20] was used in an appropriate formulation for surface TMVs, see Sect. 3.2. In both cases, electric potentials were computed on the body surface for sources of transmembrane voltages (TMVs) in the heart. For the FEM approach, an unstructured tetrahedral grid was used, which was taken care of to be a good enough representation of the cardiac sources, see specifications in Sect. 6.4. For inverse calculations, which cannot deal with numbers of unknowns in the order of the node count in the forward model, the number of heart nodes was significantly reduced. To this end, and since source gradients at mesh resolution would have geometry-induced anisotropic properties that cause artifacts, in our group, a coarse heart mesh of linear finite elements is produced and cardiac sources are interpolated on the original mesh of the heart and thorax for the forward calculation. I.e., both the shape of the heart in the original mesh as well as the structure of the reduced coarse mesh determine the representation of sources. As the forward problem of ECG is linear (linear interpolation is used between the coarse and fine grid), it can be formulated as a simple system of linear equations, represented by a lead field matrix A:

$$Ax = b. \tag{4.1}$$

The lead field matrix maps transmembrane voltages at n locations in the heart (represented as vector $x \in \mathbb{R}^{n\times 1}$) to the BSPM, which is a vector of m electrode signals $b \in \mathbb{R}^{m\times 1}$, $m << n$. To compute A, n unit vectors $\hat{x}_i$ of sources at points $i = 1 \ldots n$ in the coarse grid are interpolated from the coarse mesh on the fine grid. These sources are represented on the coarse grid in the same manner as node shape functions are defined in the finite element method (see Fig. 4.1): the TMV at one node is set to 1, and all other nodes are set to zero [21, Sect. 5.2.2]. Between the nodes, linear interpolation is used. The TMVs are interpolated in this representation on the fine grid and forward calculated, i.e. their corresponding BSPM $\hat{b}_i$ is simulated [11, Sect. 4.4.2]. As vectors $\hat{x}_i$, the single sources are linearly independent and span the space of TMVs in the coarse grid structure of the heart with the following properties (see Fig. 4.1):

$$\forall x \in \mathbb{R}^{n\times 1} : x = x_1\hat{x}_1 + x_2\hat{x}_2 + \cdots + x_n\hat{x}_n, \text{ where } x = \begin{bmatrix} x_1 \\ x_2 \\ \vdots \\ x_n \end{bmatrix} \tag{4.2}$$

$$\text{and } \hat{x}_i \in \mathbb{R}^{n\times 1} \text{ is a unit source vector, } x_{ij} = \begin{cases} 1 \; j = i \\ 0 \; j \neq i \end{cases}, \tag{4.3}$$

$$\tag{4.4}$$

see [11, Eq. 4.9]. As in a linear electric network, electrical signals from different sources combine linearly (superposition principle by Helmholtz). The BSPMs of the components in x can be weighted with the components' magnitude and combine linearly to the BSPM of x:

$$b = x_1\hat{b}_1 + x_2\hat{b}_2 + \cdots + x_n\hat{b}_n = \left[\hat{b}_1, \hat{b}_2, \ldots, \hat{b}_n\right] x := Ax \tag{4.5}$$

Note that A does not have full column rank, i.e., not all column vectors are linearly independent, and the problem of finding the source x for a given b is underdetermined. It is also ill-conditioned. The following chapter elaborates on these particular characteristics of the inverse problem of ECG.

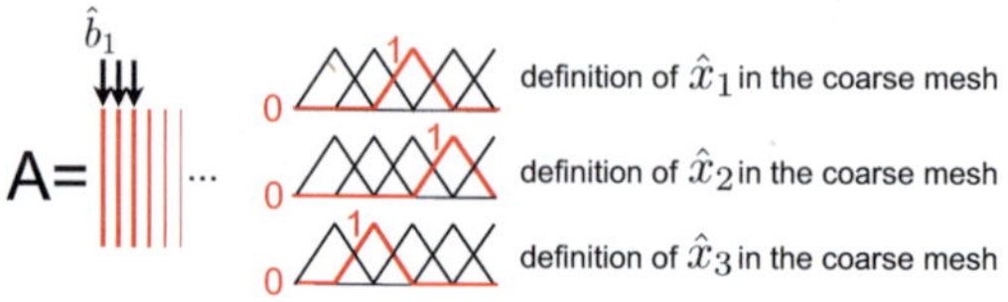

Figure 4.1: Schematic illustration of the representation of the unit vectors $\hat{x}_i$ in the coarse mesh in 1-D and their corresponding BSPMs $\hat{b}_i$ in the lead field matrix.

For calculations with the boundary element method (BEM), the lead field matrix was calculated for sources in the surface model of the endo- and epicardium directly, as the heart representation in this mesh was coarse enough to be handled by the inverse solvers. The Matlab library by Stenroos et al. [16] was used and an implementation by Danila Potyagaylo that facilitates the calculation of BSPMs from surface TMVs.

4.2 The Ill-Posedness of the Inverse Problem

The inverse problem of ECG is ill-posed according to the definition by Hadamard [22]. Although a solution for x exists (1st), it is neither unique (2nd) nor does the solution depend continuously on the given data (3rd criterion):

The aforementioned underdeterminedness leads to multiple solutions being possible. For transmembrane voltages, the offset in x is arbitrary and within the null space of A, as only gradients in x cause a BSPM. Another example are sources in the septum. While Fig. 4.2a shows an excitation wavefront that started from the red bullet (epicardium of the LV) and is correctly reconstructed with a Tikhonov solver, the TMV distribution in Fig. 4.2b is clearly reconstructed with the greatest voltages at the lateral wall of the RV. I.e., while the BSPM was produced for an excitation origin in the septum, the given solution produces the same BSPM with a source in the lateral wall.

On top of that, mathematical solvers have to deal with the strong attenuation of cardiac signals by the body. This is especially true for cardiac signals of high spatial frequency and represented in the decay of singular values of A, which is shown in Fig. 4.3. While low spatial frequencies tend to be mapped to the BSPM with great singular values σ_i, it is commonly the case that for the higher spatial frequencies, much smaller singular values apply (condition numbers reflect this ratio and are in the order of, e.g., 10^8 for lead field matrices). Eigenvectors in the singular value decomposition are not only ordered by the magnitude of their singular values, but according to [24, 2.2.1] also tend to have more zero-crossings along with smaller magnitudes, i.e. greater spatial frequency (this behaviour is often observed for discrete ill-posed problems in general). As high frequency source components experience strong damping (small singular values), the corresponding BSPM components must be strongly amplified to reconstruct the related cardiac source components. This amplification is of such high magnitude that any noise in the BSPM easily corrupts the solution, up to the extent of being sensitive to the effects of finite numerical precision [25]. To reduce the discontinuous behaviour of the solution, ECG imaging usually only images the cardiac activity up to a relatively low resolution, which is achieved through regularization of the solution.

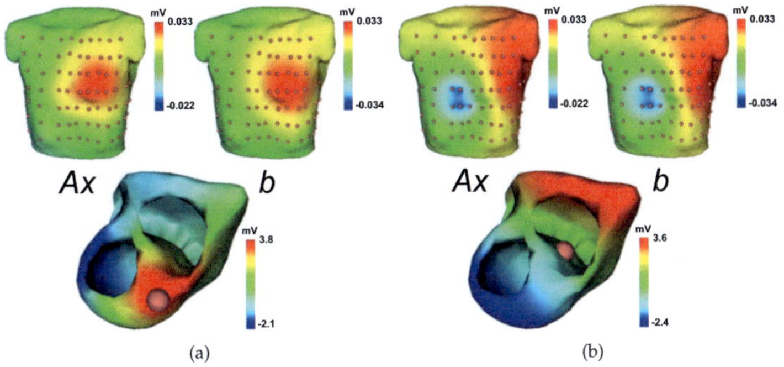

Figure 4.2: Solutions to $x = \underset{x}{\operatorname{argmin}} \|Ax - b\|_2^2 + \lambda^2 \|Lx\|_2^2$, $\lambda = 10^{-2}$, for an ectopic beat simulated at the epicardium of the LV (a) and for an excitation origin (red bullet) that is simulated at the septum of the RV (b). Whereas in (a) the right location is found, in (b) a wrong solution is reconstructed. Figure adapted from presentation in [23].

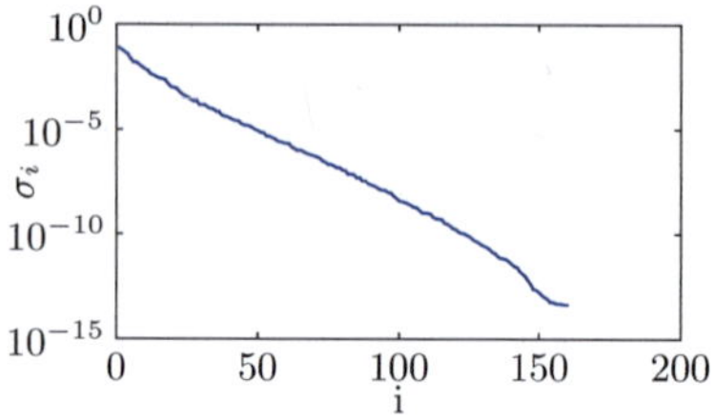

Figure 4.3: Decay of singular values σ_i in A for a thorax model with 160 electrodes; adapted from [26], where the behaviour was studied for clinical electrode setups.

4.3 Regularization Techniques

For a system of linear equations $Ax = b$, a solution x_M can be found that either has the minimum squared L2 norm of the residual

$$\forall x: \; \|Ax - b\|_2^2 > \|Ax_M - b\|_2^2 \tag{4.6}$$

or the minimum squared L2 norm among those x that produce equality in the previous term (for underdetermined systems)

$$x_M = \underset{x}{\operatorname{argmin}} \|x\|_2^2 \; s.t. \; \|Ax - b\|_2^2 = \|Ax_M - b\|_2^2. \tag{4.7}$$

The solution $x_M = A^\dagger$ can be proven to solve the problem, where $A^\dagger$ is the Moore-Penrose pseudo-inverse [27, Eq. 5]. $A^\dagger$ can be expressed as a simple algebraic formula in the case of A having full row or full column rank. According to [28, Eq. 9], in the case of full row rank (which is a characteristic of A unless electrodes are really close to one another), $A^\dagger$ can be computed from the singular vectors u_i and v_i of $A = U\Sigma V^T$ as $A^\dagger = \sum_{i_1}^{\text{rank}(A)} u_i^T \frac{1}{\sigma_i} v_i$. Despite delivering unique solutions with minimum norm in the second case (and hence coping with the 2nd criterion of ill-posedness), the singular value decomposition clearly reveals that the solution is still subject to the ill-conditioned nature of the problem, i.e. small singular values in the reciprocal term lead to a great amplification of high-frequency components in the data. To produce a solution that is stable against high-frequency noise, regularization is required.

4.3.1 Tikhonov Regularization (Tikh)

To the end of imposing smoothness on the solution of the inverse problem (Tikhonov regularization, Tikh) and to thereby stabilizing the results, a regularization term $||Lx||_2^2$ is added to the residual [29].

$$x = \underset{x}{\operatorname{argmin}} ||Ax - b||_2^2 + \lambda^2 ||Lx||_2^2 \tag{4.8}$$

$$\Leftrightarrow x = \underset{x}{\operatorname{argmin}} (Ax - b)^T (Ax - b) + \lambda^2 (Lx)^T (Lx) \tag{4.9}$$

The cost functional is convex, i.e., its extremum is also its minimum. With some basic algebra from [30], this yields:

$$\Leftrightarrow 0 = 2A^T(Ax - b) + 2\lambda^2 L^T Lx \tag{4.10}$$

$$\Leftrightarrow 0 = (A^T A + \lambda^2 L^T L)x - A^T b \tag{4.11}$$

$$\Leftrightarrow x = (A^T A + \lambda^2 L^T L)^{-1} A^T b, \tag{4.12}$$

where L is a discrete approximation of the Laplace operator (in case of 2nd order Tikhonov) and λ is the regularization parameter, which is challenging to optimize due to its strong influence on the solution. The L-curve method [31] was implemented to select the best λ in this work, unless a specific choice is explicitly stated. Its implementation follows the algorithms in the Matlab toolbox by Hansen [32]. The latter implementation fits a 2-D spline curve to the smoothed discrete L-curve. It then locates the point on the discrete L-curve which is closest to its corner.

Note that, in order to find a closed-form solution, the problem was stated in this case as a least-squares problem with squared L2 norm components and a squared regularization parameter λ^2. Many algorithms in this work are defined and implemented with functionals that have un-squared λ parameters and/or L2 norms, i.e. the appropriate parameter ranges and effects of the norms on the cost balancing must be considered for each method individually.

4.3.2 Tikhonov-Greensite Regularization (TikhGS)

While Tikhonov regularization performs smoothing in space, it treats all time steps separately in its basic formulation. The spatio-temporal Tikhonov method by Greensite [33] (TikhGS) approaches the problem through the temporal domain as well and imposes temporal smoothness by reducing the information in the ECG to its most relevant singular vectors in time (which automatically leads to a reduction of the spatial information as well). This has the beautiful side-effect of the signal being reduced to its major components, which minimizes the time of computation for cardiac source time sequences. The approach is easily formulated as follows:

$$AX = B = USV^T, \tag{4.13}$$

$X = [x_1 \cdots x_T]$, $B = [b_1 \cdots b_T]$, where T: length of the BSPM time frame.

$$\Leftrightarrow A(XV) = US \tag{4.14}$$

The forward problem is now formulated with the BSPM represented by its singular vectors in time. The time samples in that singular vector representation are reduced to $1 \dots p$ components. As guideline for choosing parameter p, the finding in [34] may be consulted which suggests that 11 singular vectors in time are sufficient to represent a BSPM. Alternatively, an automatic scheme was proposed by Greensite, see [11, Eq. 4.39].
The inverse problem is now solved after (XV) using the Tikhonov method,

$$(XV)_\lambda = \underset{(XV)}{\operatorname{argmin}} \|A(XV) - US\|_2^2 + \lambda^2 \|L(XV)\|_2^2, \tag{4.15}$$

and the result multiplied with $V^T \in \mathbb{R}^{p \times T}$ to transform back to the solution X in time.

Note that the presented notation follows that of [21, Sect. 5.3.8], which can be proven to be equivalent to its documentation in [33] and [11, Sect. 4.6.5] and again to that of the proposed method in Sect. 5.4. Regularization parameter λ was chosen using the L-curve method as proposed in [31], including smoothing and 2-D interpolation.

4.3.3 Maximum A-Posteriori Method (MAP)

The maximum a-posteriori (MAP) method facilitates regularization of the Tikhonov-based inverse solution in space based on a priori statistical information that may be obtained from simulations of cardiac excitation propagation, namely the covariance of the sources' spatial distribution. The method has been proposed in [35] and was used in [36, 37] with the support of then improved models of cardiac excitation propagation. It is derived as follows, in line with the presentation in [38, 5.4.6] and [39]: Let e be the measurement error in

$$b = Ax + e \tag{4.16}$$

In oder to obtain an optimal solution of the problem, a solution estimate $\hat{x}$ is proposed for Eq. 4.16,

$$\hat{x} = Hb \tag{4.17}$$

$$\Leftrightarrow \hat{x} = HAx + He, \tag{4.18}$$

where x and e are assumed to have zero mean.
The estimation error of $\hat{x}$ leads to two summands

$$\hat{x} - x = (HA - I)x + He \tag{4.19}$$

where the first term represents the error of H in solving Ax after x, i.e. its capability of solving the inverse problem, while the second term represents the measurement error, which is mapped to the space of x. According to [39, Eq. 20] the covariance of this error can be calculated as

$$C = (HA - I)C_x(HA - I)^T + HC_eH^T, \tag{4.20}$$

assuming that the sought solution x varies with respect to its zero mean by a supposedly known covariance of C_x and the measurement error e, which is assumed to be statistically independent, by a covariance of C_e. Minimization after H yields the minimum variance estimator:

$$H = C_x A^T (A C_x A^T + C_e)^{-1} \tag{4.21}$$

By inserting H into Eq. 4.17, the inverse problem can now be solved optimally, given the measurement and estimate error covariances, yielding

$$\hat{x} = Hb = C_x A^T (A C_x A^T + C_e)^{-1} b \tag{4.22}$$

To obtain an estimate of C_x, simulations of cardiac excitation propagation were performed with samples of x collected in a stochastical basis $S = [x_1 x_2 \ldots x_N]$ and C_x computed as

$$C_x = \frac{1}{N}(S - \overline{S})(S - \overline{S})^T, \tag{4.23}$$

where $\overline{S}$ is the mean of S.
To this end, ectopic beats were started from every 3rd node in the ventricles and a sample of x was taken at a specific time in the beat (a good choice for this time of sampling is studied in Sect. 7.1.2). For both BEM and FEM models, a variant of the fastest route algorithm was implemented as presented in the works of van Dam et al. [40], yet with isotropic and homogeneous excitation conduction velocities. The Dijkstra algorithm was used to compute distances between the cardiac nodes through shortest paths in the mesh, and connectivities were taken from the Laplace operator in FEM. In BEM, based on the work of Danila Potyagaylo and Vynnie Kong, such connectivity matrices were produced also for surface meshes, including surface-to-surface links. Two spatio-temporal variants of the MAP approach were implemented as well, which produce results with the Greensite spatio-temporal approach from Sect. 4.3.2 either for the entire QRS (MAPSTqrs) or a win-

dow around the time to be evaluated (MAPSTwin), all with the number of considered eigenvectors in the BSPM set to $p = 10$, in line with the finding in [11, 34]. Accordingly, additional samples were added to S in the calculation of C_x, one for each time sample in the domain of eigenvectors, i.e. for each 3rd node p samples were introduced to the stochastical basis. Especially for the FEM method, it was not feasible to consider beats from each point in the mesh for the sheer size of the matrix to be processed, and the number of samples was considered great enough to parameterize C_x.
C_e was approximated by a diagonal matrix that was further simplified to a weighted identy matrix $C_e = \varepsilon I$, where ε can be considered a regularization parameter. C_e could theoretically be computed from the measurement noise and from modeling errors in A, should they be Gaussian in b. These errors are not known. However, ε could be found to lead to an L-curve-like behaviour in $\|AXV - BV\|_2$ over $\|C_x XV\|_2$ (spectral norms), the latter of which is the similarity of the results to the covariance matrix. The choice of ε was made using a smoothed and interpolated L-curve with the toolbox by Hansen [32].

4.3.4 Activation Time Imaging Based on the TMV Time Integral (ATintT2)

The time integral of TMVs over the QRS can be linked to the underlying activation times. This effect has been studied within the scope of this work [41] and is illustrated in Fig. 4.4. The time integral of the TMVs x between 0 ms and T ms, corresponding to $k = 1 \dots k_T$ in samples with sampling interval t_s, can be approximated as:

$$\tilde{x} := \int_0^T x\,dt \approx t_s \sum_{k=1}^{k_T} x_k. \tag{4.24}$$

Given a healthy action potential in a component in $x(t)$ (see blue curve in the upper left plot in Fig. 4.4), the integral of the component between 0 and T ms is a falling curve over k_T which stops to fall as soon as the action potential depolarizes, see blue curve in the lower left plot. I.e., when integrating over the entire QRS ($k_T = 101$) in the healthy case, which is depicted in the first column, large TMV integrals are of action potentials with early depolarization, small TMV integrals correspond to very late depolarizations. The unit of these TMV integrals is mVms. Mathematically, the finding leads to a linear formulation of the forward problem that can be used for activation time imaging as proposed in [38, 42]. When defining $\tilde{x}$ as integral over the entire QRS interval $t = 0 \dots T_{qrs}$ now, then

$$\tilde{x} := \int_0^{T_{qrs}} x\,dt \approx t_s \sum_{k=1}^{k_{T_{qrs}}} x_k. \tag{4.25}$$

With linearity in $Ax = b$ follows that

$$A\tilde{x} = t_s \sum_{k=1}^{k_{T_{qrs}}} Ax_k = t_s \sum_{k=1}^{k_{T_{qrs}}} b_k := \tilde{b}. \tag{4.26}$$

I.e., when computing the sum of all BSPM samples in the QRS

$$\tilde{b} = t_s \sum_{k=1}^{k_{T_{qrs}}} b_k. \tag{4.27}$$

the problem $A\tilde{x} = \tilde{b}$ can be solved after $\tilde{x}$ with the Tikhonov method, yielding TMV-integrals over the QRS as displayed in the lower plots of Fig. 4.4:

$$\tilde{x}_{\mathrm{ATintT2}} = \underset{\tilde{x}}{\operatorname{argmin}} \left\{ \|A\tilde{x} - \tilde{b}\|_2 + \lambda^2 \|L\tilde{x}\|_2 \right\}, \tag{4.28}$$

where L is the Laplace operator and λ chosen using the L-curve method [31] with the corner detection algorithm by Hansen [32], including smoothing and spline interpolation.

Assuming that all TMV action potentials have identical shapes, the TMV-integral over the QRS may be interpreted as an activation sequence, given that the action potential curve is weakly increasing. Note that this is a general finding which distinguishes the work in [42] from previous articles [43]. These had proposed the use of TMV time-integrals as well, but imposed models on the TMV action potentials such as a Heaviside function [25] or arctan-function [44].

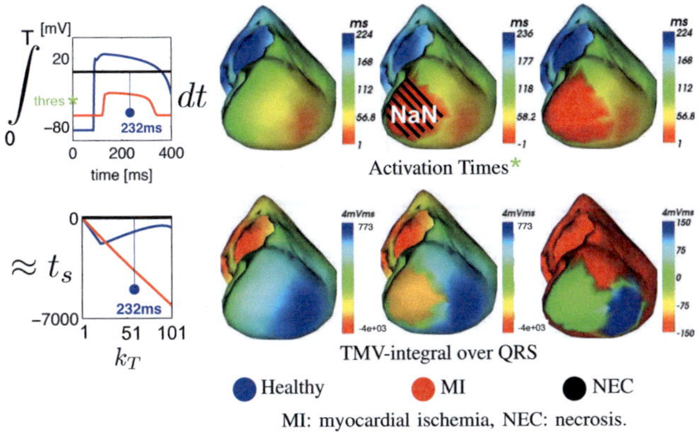

Figure 4.4: The time integral of TMVs over the QRS can be linked to their underlying activation times (see simulation of a healthy PVC beat, blue). Lines in the upper plot show typical action potential curves, the lower plot demonstrates how the areas under the curves evolve over time, excluding the sampling time factor. The same is also demonstrated for a PVC with an area of myocardial ischemia (MI) and necrosis (NEC). Figures adapted from [41]. Blue (healthy), red (MI) and black (NEC) colors correspond to the curves in the plots. For MI, the affected region is classified as NaN (-1).

The integral method is used without further interpretation or normalization of the TMV time-integral in this work, as it is only used for imaging of activation origins. While taking advantage of the fact that solutions are valid for any continuously increasing action potential shape, it must be noted that for physiological action potentials, the latter requirement is violated. However, despite being a correct assumption for the mathematics in [42] to hold, it is not the minimum requirement: to have an activation sequence represented in the results, it is still sufficient to have an action potential shape with continuously increasing TMV time integral (after depolarization), which is shown to be true for the morphology presented in Fig. 4.4 for the healthy case (blue). Later on, for activation time imaging, a Heaviside assumption is made for the action potentials, see Sect. 5.3, which also presents a new modification of this approach.

It was found in the clinical studies at King's College London that scars lead to artifacts of homogeneous areas in the solutions for TMV time integrals. The study in [41] demonstrates that this is indeed the case, using action potential shapes of ischemic (MI) scar from [45] and — for comparison, a TMV level for necrotic (NEC) tissue of 0 mV as proposed in [37]. Simulations in Fig. 4.4 show that early activation times produce homogeneous areas of low (MI) or medium (NEC) time-integrals indeed, leading to an interpretation of these areas as late activation times. This effect is also reflected in the inverse solutions of Fig. 4.5, where the the results with the ATintT2 method have been converted to activation times.

> Note: From the TMV integral the activation time can be calculated if the action potential is known. If it is not known, it can still be interpreted as activation sequence, but in the unit mVms, and with large values representing early activation.

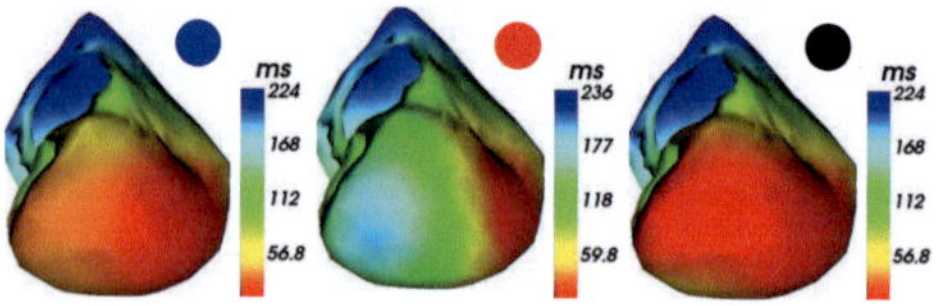

Figure 4.5: ECG imaging results with the ATintT2 method for BSPMs from the simulated activation sequences in Fig. 4.4. The TMV integral has been converted to activation times using the assumption of a Heaviside function. Figures are adapted from [41].

4.3.5 Approach of Reconstructing Critical Points and Times (CritT)

A well-posed formulation of the inverse problem of computing activation times was found in 1994 by Fred Greensite [46], under the assumption that action potentials have the behaviour of step functions. The method was validated for the first time by Greensite and Huiskamp in 1997 [47]. Using "jump maps" and an approach derived from the MUltiple SIgnal Classification (MUSIC) algorithm in antenna theory, it can reliably produce activation times (critical times) for the spatial extrema of activation time maps (critical points).
Critical points are singularities of $M_0^T(i)$, where $M_0^k(i)$ is

$$M_0^k(i) = \left| 1 - \sum_{r=1}^{r_{eff}} \langle \alpha_i, U_r^{[0,k]} \rangle^2 \right|^{-1} \tag{4.29}$$

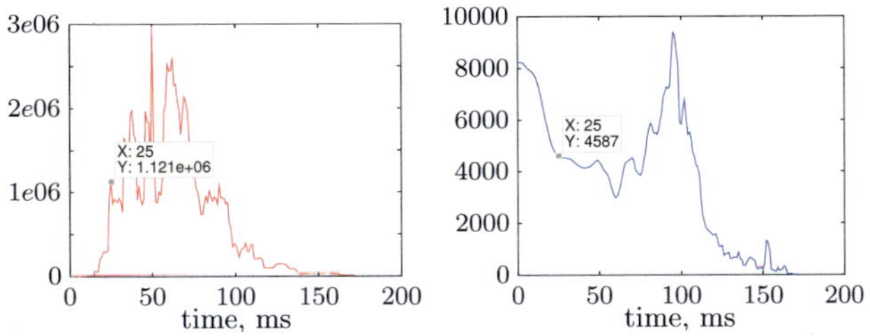

(a) $M^+(i = 1325)$ (b) $M^-(i = 1325)$

Figure 4.6: The distance of the BSPM of a cardiac node to the most important spatial components of the measured BSPM signal is represented in these functions for the time from the start of the QRS (a) and up to the end of the QRS (b) (node $i = 1325$ depolarizes at 25 ms).

and

$$\sum_{r=1}^{r_{eff}} \langle \alpha_i, U_r^{[0,k]} \rangle^2 \tag{4.30}$$

are the distances between the i-th column a_i of the leadfield matrix A, which is the BSPM of the respective node i in the heart, and the $r = 1 \ldots r_{\mathrm{eff}}$ spatial singular vectors $U_r^{[0,k]}$ of the measured BSPM B. For the distance to be computed, the singular value decomposition computes these spatial characteristics from the interval specified in upper and lower indices of $M_0^k(i)$, i.e. $B^{[0,k]} = [b_0, \ldots, b_k] = U^{[0,k]} S^{[0,k]} V^{[0,k]}$. a_i is normalized to $\alpha_i = \frac{a_i}{\|a_i\|_2^2}$ for comparison with the unit vectors in U, and k may be any time step in the BSPM of the QRS complex $k = 1 \ldots T$.
While critical points $M_0^T(i)$ are hence computed from the BSPM of the entire QRS, an interesting behaviour of $M_0^k(i)$ can be used to calculate activation times for critical points: when computing the distance measure of a source i to the BSPM $M_0^k(i)$ for different times k it makes a significant upstroke at the time of its depolarization. This effect is used to compute the activation times of critical points and illustrated in Fig. 4.6a for a heart node that depolarizes at 25 ms.
To identify the significant upstroke, a method is proposed in [47, Sect. II] that computes not only the distance to the singular vectors of the BSPM up to a point of time in $M^+(i,k) = M_0^k(i)$, but also takes into account how well a source is represented in the BSPM that follows the current

time step $M^-(i,k) = M_k^T(i)$. Naturally, $M^+(i,k)$ tends to increase after depolarization of a source (Fig. 4.6a) and $M^-(i,k)$ tends to decrease (Fig. 4.6b). Subtracting $M^-(i,k)$ from $M^+(i,k)$ yields a function

$$Z(i,k) = M^+(i,k) - M^-(i,k) \tag{4.31}$$

that has a zero-crossing near the critical time of a critical point i — and that also has the strongest jump at the critical time for a critical point. Computing activation times by identification of these zero-crossings is called the critical times method (CritT). The derivation of the method assumes that action potentials have the behaviour of a Heaviside function in time, which is a good approximation for the time of the QRS. The method is proven in [47] to work for critical points on the heart surface under this assumption. Times produced for surface points that lie between critical points can be considered interpolations of the activation times of the critical points according to the paper. In this work, the method is used only for the BEM method, but it could well be used to reconstruct activation times in the myocardial volume as well, which can be interpreted as another extension of the interpolation.

4.4 State-of-the-Art

Several review papers are available as introductions to the inverse problem of electrocardiography. Table 4.1 provides a collection of review papers, including reviews also on the forward calculation and a paper that describes in detail the entire processing workflow for solving the inverse problem of ECG.

The field of ECG imaging is currently undergoing a phase of great attention in both the clinical and technical field. Two companies have started to commercialize systems for solving the inverse problem of ECG. First, CardioInsight Technologies Inc. from Cleveland, OH in the United States, which is a company that started as a spin-off with people from the group of Yoram Rudy [58, 59]. The company holds several international patents and its technology is well published by key cardiologists, see e.g. a review article on the technology by Michel Haissaguerre

Author(s)	Topic	Reference
Seger, Pfeifer, Berger	Entire workflow, maths: ECG imaging	[48]
Oosterom	Inverse problem of bioelectricity	[49]
Pullan, Cheng, Nash, Ghodrati, MacLeod, Brooks	Inverse problem of ECG	[50]
Dössel	Inverse problem of ECG and MCG	[51]
Gulrajani	Inverse problem of ECG	[52]
Brooks, MacLeod	Inverse problem of ECG	[53]
Brooks, MacLeod	Inverse problem of ECG	[54]
Oosterom	Inverse problem of ECG	[55]
Johnson	Bioelectric field calculation	[56]
Greensite	ECG imaging: mathematical basis	[14]
Gulrajani	Modeling and simulation for ECG imaging	[57]

Table 4.1: Reviews and introductions to ECG imaging, with the latest publications listed first.

et al. [60]. Second, EP Solutions SA from Yverdon-les-Bains, Switzerland. The company originally operated under the name AMYCARD LLC which is located in Moscow, Russia. It also holds international patents [61], works with physicians that have recently published abstracts [62] on a comparison of results against a 64-electrode basket catheter of the FIRMap system by Topera, Inc., Menlo Park, CA, USA. EP Solutions has published several works on their system [63] and its mathematics [64].

Little is known about the technology of the commercial ECG imaging methods. However, the abstract [62] clearly reveals that the EP Solutions system uses epicardial mapping in the presented work, neglecting the endocardium. The same is pointed out in [63], where the method used by the scientists of EP Solutions is presented as mapping electrograms either at the endocardial surface or at the epicardium. This supports an argument in [65] that claims that current commercial systems use either endocardial mapping or epicardial mapping for ECG imaging, but not both, depending on the location of the probe. A work by Rudy et al. [66] is given as a reference for the claim, which images epicardial potentials only. The same holds true for the most-cited publication of the group [59] and for the validation study listed below [67].

The goal of the present study was to perform and validate ECG imaging in humans, with the objective of improving interventional treatment planning for radio-frequency ablation procedures. In the context of existing studies, which have deployed methods for the reconstruction of extracellular potentials [66, 67] or surface activation times [68, 69], the approach in this work was to use transmembrane voltages (TMVs) as the underlying source model.

For TMVs, validation in humans is to date only possible for activation times. Or in the case of localizing the origin of a premature ventricular contraction (PVC), it is possible to validate the ability to localize the PVC focus. Both has been done in this study. Compared to extracellular potentials, TMVs better visualize the real areas of activation and at the same time serve as a physiology-related interface for introducing a-priori knowledge into the solutions of the inverse problem of ECG. Their transmural visualization (given very accurate models) allows for direct physiological interpretation.

Conventional non-invasive imaging modalities provide only insufficient guidance for ablation therapies [70], which require long-lasting catheter measurements during therapy. The goal of this work was therefore to proove and push the capabilities of ECG imaging to a level where it facilitates accurate therapy planning. In addition, a goal of this work was to test whether it is possible to enhance invasively measured electro-anatomical maps with pre-interventionally collected data, especially for cases with little arrhythmic activity.

To give an overview of ECG imaging validation studies performed so far in humans, Table 4.2 is made that lists the source models with emphasis on the imaged surfaces, characterizes the cases, and cites the related publications.

Reviews	Reference
Validation studies of ECGI: approaches, history and state	[50] Macfarlane et al.
Validation studies of ECGI: challenges	[71] Nash & Pullan

Source model	Cases	Reference
EP (epicardium)	9 patients imaged during sustained VT, localization error: qualitative agreement CARTO endocardial validation	[66] Wang & Rudy
EP (epicardium)	localization error of pacing cites: $\approx 1\,\text{cm}$ open chest surgery, intraoperative epicardial mapping with two 100-electrode patches	[67] Ghanem & Rudy
EP (epicardium)	RBBB, left and right ventricular pacing, chronic atrial flutter; localization error: qualitative agreement	[59] Ramanathan & Rudy
EP (epicardium)	single PVC, localization error: imaged and measured activation origins "correlated", CARTO endocardial and epicardial validation (epicardial ablation via xiphoid puncture)	[72] Intini & Rudy
EP (epicardium)	11-23 epicardial pacing sites in 4 patients, mean localization error: $13-28\,\text{mm}$ in areas without scar and $28-67\,\text{mm}$ in areas of scar or in the scar margin CARTO epicardial validation	[73] Sapp & Horácek
EP (epicardium)	VT: clinically identified exit sites or successful ablation sites of two out of six induced VTs, localization error: qualitative agreement; no activation sequences recorded. CARTO epicardial validation	[73] Sapp & Horácek
EP (endo- and epicardium)	ventricles, 3 patients, imprecise thorax model, 1000+ pacings, mean localization error $3-5\,\text{cm}$, CARTO validation	[65] Erem & Brooks
AT (endo- and epicardium)	WPW pathway: excitation origin, mean localization error 19 mm CARTO endocardial validation	[74] Berger & Tilg
AT (endo- and epicardium)	atria, pacing CS, SN; localization error $6-12\text{mm}$, CARTO endocardial validation	[68] Tilg et al.
AT (endo- and epicardium)	atria, pacing RAA, CS, high RA; localization error $8-14\text{mm}$, CARTO endocardial validation	[75] Hanser & Tilg
AT (endo- and epicardium)	atria, pacings, localization error $\leq 10\,\text{mm}$ CARTO endocardial validation	[76] Modre & Tilg
ECD (endocardium)	PVC, last ablation site, localization error: $13.8 \pm 1.3\text{mm}$	[77] Lai & He
ESMD	PVC, last ablation site, localization error: $25.5 \pm 5.5\text{mm}$	[77] Lai & He
EP (epicardium)	localization of acute MI from occlusions produced by angioplasty balloon inflation during percutaneous transluminal coronary angioplasty (PTCA), localization error: qualitative agreement	[78] MacLeod & Horácek

Table 4.2: ECG Imaging human validation studies. AT: surface activation times, EP: extracellular potentials, ECD: equivalent current density, ESMD: equivalent single moving dipole, RBBB: right bundle branch block.

5

Proposed Methods for Solving the Inverse Problem of ECG

"Don't think, just act."

Peter van Dam

In addition to applying existing techniques, new approaches have been proposed for solving the inverse problem of ECG: variants of state-space approaches that introduce models of cardiac excitation propagation in inverse solutions for stabilization, improved approaches for imaging activation times, including a framework that makes inverse calculations available to augment measurements in invasive procedures with data from non-invasive pre-interventional recordings. Further, an approach is presented that solves the signal processing problem of removing the offset in the BSPM within the context of the inverse problem of ECG, and a simple model-based approach is presented, albeit for documentation of its implementation rather than its novelty.

5.1 State Space Models

The inverse problem of ECG is severely ill-posed, but a lot is known about the cardiac excitation spread. This knowledge cannot easily be represented in linear terms, and hence it is very difficult to introduce it in linearly formulated optimization problems. This has motivated the use of model-based solvers [79–83] that use optimization approaches for non-linear models to fine-tune their parameters, intending them to converge in a solution that reflects the actual excitation spread in the heart. The problem of these solvers is the rigidity of their models, i.e. their inability to adapt to pathological conditions, correct for modeling errors — or otherwise their great dimensionality in case of taking such aspects into account.

In the pursuit of introducing as much a-priori knowledge in the solution as possible, while leaving room for its physiological and pathological variations, this work has started from the idea of introducing a recursive state space model of the cardiac excitation propagation in a Kalman filter [84] that would be used to introduce a-priori knowledge from the model in a data-driven solution of the inverse problem. As the cardiac excitation behaviour depends strongly on the offset of the solution when represented in terms of TMVs, the challenge of working within the loop of a recursive Kalman filter, state estimates were not produced in a physiological range. This is due to the forward problem, which is

used by the Kalman filter to correct state estimates against the error they cause in the BSPM, not taking into account offsets in the source, as they are in the null space of the lead field matrix.
The initial approach was first to study how physiological levels can be induced in the inverse solutions for linear formulations, leading to a "range-adjusted Tikhonov method" which was shown to work well with a recursive cellular automaton [85]. Results were shown to depend strongly on the excitation conduction velocity used for the parameterization of the automaton, i.e. the approach was unlikely to leave enough room for the data to correct the model. As a first step, it still served as a template on how recursive models could be introduced in the Kalman filter — and it proposed a method for keeping the solution in a physiological range. A Kalman filter with augmented measurement model was then introduced [86], where the augmented measurements represent the regularization term of the linear inverse problem. This implementation allows for an explicit regularization of the Kalman filter estimate. However, in the initial implementation shown in the paper, a linear prediction model was chosen and parameterized as simply as possible to reveal the effects of the covariance matrices and their parameterization. Results made clear that despite the augmented measurement model being a good format of introducing regularization, a non-linear system model must be used to effectively handle the inverse problem of imaging TMVs in a state-space framework. This was the motivation to use an unscented Kalman filter algorithm, which is used to handle non-linear models and had previously been applied in ECG imaging by Wang et al. [87], yet with a reaction-diffusion model [88]. The focus was to study the nonlinear model related effects, not the effects of the solution range of the state estimate on the propagation. Therefore, the filter was designed to process range-constrained solutions of the inverse problem directly instead of solving the inverse problem and processing BSPMs, which are usually regarded as the measurements in existing works with Kalman filters. The purpose of the filter was to improve the solutions' accuracy and to clean them from artifacts. For the purpose of specifying the solution range, after an initial approach published in [85],

a well-performing method [89] appeared at that time, which was used then to produce the input data for the filter. Results with the unscented Kalman filter are currently being documented, but are beyond the scope of this thesis. Future applications of the filter might get back to another idea presented earlier in the context of this work, which is the tolerance operator that reduces regularization along the wave front [90]. Instead of a homogeneous model for the system noise covariance, it may serve as a feature for a region-specific training of the noise covariance matrix.

5.2 Sigmoid Weighting in Critical Times Activation Time Imaging

Fig. 4.6 in Sect. 4.3.5 reveals that the functions in which the most important spatial components of the measured BSPM signal are represented for the time from the start of the QRS up to a given point in time $M^+(i,k)$ (Fig. 4.6a) and from a given point in time up to the end of the QRS (Fig. 4.6b) may have significant differences in magnitude. The derivation in [47, Sect. II] reveals that function $Z(p,k) = M^+(i,k) - M^-(i,k)$ from Eq. 4.31 is a feature that tends to lead to zero-crossings at the critical time, but it is not a strict feature. The only strict feature in the function $Z(i,k)$ is that its strongest upstroke is exactly at the critical time given i is a critical point [47]. Therefore, $Z(i,k)$ is heuristically defined and may be adapted using heuristic approaches as well without violating the theory behind the method in [47].

We observed that given the extreme differences in magnitude even the slightest noise in $M^+(i,k)$ of Fig. 4.6a can easily top the magnitude of $M^-(i,k)$ in (Fig. 4.6b). This motivated a leveling of the magnitudes with a sigmoid function. It would suppress small signals and cause an almost linear behaviour for medium magnitudes that would leave the shape of the functions mostly untouched.

Let the maximum value of M^+ and the initial value of M^- be defined as

$$\max(M^+) := \max(M^+(i,[1:T])) \tag{5.1}$$

$$\text{init}(M^-) := M^-(i,1). \tag{5.2}$$

The correction is performed for each node i individually:

$$Z_{\text{sigmoid}}(i,k) = \frac{\max(M^+)}{1+e^{-a(M^+(i,k)-s)}} - M^-(i,k), \tag{5.3}$$

where the origin of the sigmoid function $\frac{1}{1+e^{-x}}$ is shifted to

$$s = \sigma_s \max(M^+) \tag{5.4}$$

and a is chosen such that at $\frac{1}{15}\max(M^+)$ the left term in Eq. 5.3 is as low as $\frac{1}{10}\text{init}(M^-)$, which determines the steepness of the sigmoid function in $Z_{\text{sigmoid}}(i,k)$.

$$\frac{\max(M^+)}{1+e^{-a(\frac{1}{15}\max(M^+)-s)}} = \frac{1}{10}\text{init}(M^-) \tag{5.5}$$

$$\Leftrightarrow a = -\frac{\log\left(\frac{\max(M^+)}{\frac{1}{10}\text{init}(M^-)} - 1\right)}{\frac{1}{15}\max(M^+) - s}, \tag{5.6}$$

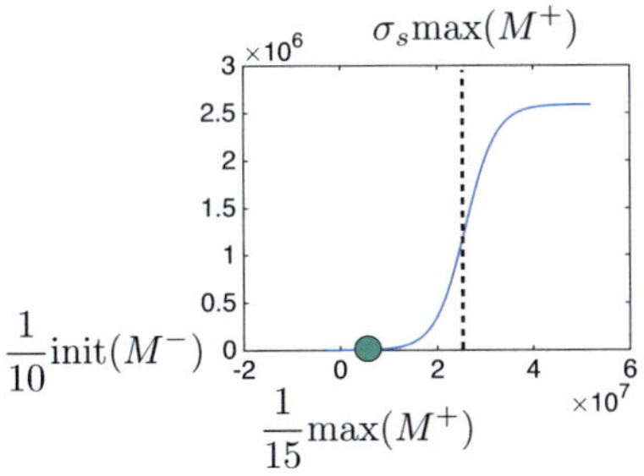

Figure 5.1: Illustration of the parameters in Eq. 5.3 to Eq. 5.6.

The method may be framed as a heuristic approach of suppressing noise in $M^+(i,k)$. It served the reconstruction results of activation time imaging in the atria impressively for the simulation study in [91] (root mean squared errors reduced from 35 ms down to between 25 ms and 20 ms for a wide range of $\sigma_s \in [10, 40]$). However, in the presence of 30 dB white Gaussian noise, similar improvements were seen, which were due only to the presence of noise, and the improvement by the sigmoid weighting was maintained only for a narrow range of σ_s, while it worsened results for the other values. The effect of the noise can be explained with a smoother interpolation between activation times at critical points. White noise is already stated in [47] as imposing a gradual offset between reconstructed critical times. As the improvements were very significant (both those through the noise and those through the weighting method), further studies on the effect of noise conditions on the interpolation could greatly improve the practical value of the critical times method for activation time imaging. From knowledge on the magnitudes and shapes of the similarity functions under such conditions, the circumstances and parameterizations could be derived for the approach to being beneficial also under realistic conditions.

5.3 A Framework to Introduce Measurements into Solutions of Activation Time Imaging

The following scheme is proposed to image activation times, given that single measurements of local activation times (LATs) in the heart are available, which is the case for the datasets in the PVC validation study. This method may serve in the future to use pre-interventional BSPM and MRI recordings to enhance sparse LAT maps, which cardiologist often have to deal with when patient arrhythmias under treatment show little activity in the catheter lab. This often leads to the termination of long-planned and stressful interventions.

The method is based on activation time imaging using the integral method and Tikhonov 2nd-order regularization (ATintT2, see Sect. 4.3.4), which was proposed and studied in [38, 41–43], where it was shown that the time integral of TMVs can be interpreted as activation sequence — or in terms of activation times when making specific assumptions on the action potential shape.

Assuming that during the QRS complex, TMVs behave like a Heaviside function in time that is scaled with Δv, it can be shown that [38]

$$A\tau = \tilde{b}, \tag{5.7}$$

where τ is the activation time and A the lead field matrix

$$\tilde{b} = -\frac{t_s}{\Delta v}\sum_{k=1}^{k_T} b_k \tag{5.8}$$

the scaled time integral of the BSPM with sampling interval t_s and BSPM time samples b_k. A solution for τ can be obtained using Tikhonov 2nd-order regularization

$$\tau_\lambda = \underset{\tau}{\operatorname{argmin}} \|A\tau - \tilde{b}\|_2 + \lambda^2 \|L\tau\|_2, \tag{5.9}$$

where L is the discrete approximation of the Laplace operator and λ the regularization parameter, which is obtained from the smoothed and interpolated L-curve using the toolbox from [32]. Solutions with the method do usually not have the correct scale and differ from that of the ground truth due to imprecise assumptions being made for Δv. However, it is possible to correct for errors in Δv even after solving the problem. Given, e.g., that a solution τ has vector entries from 0 to 140 ms, but it is known to represent the activation times of an entire QRS duration of 0 to 100 ms, it may be deduced from τ being wrong by a factor of $\alpha = 1.4$ that $1/\Delta v$ had been wrong by a factor of $\alpha = 1.4$, since for an arbitrary $\alpha \in \mathbb{R}$:

$$\underset{\tau}{\operatorname{argmin}} \|A\alpha\tau - \alpha\tilde{b}\|_2 + \lambda^2 \|L\alpha\tau\|_2 \tag{5.10}$$

$$= \underset{\tau}{\operatorname{argmin}} |\alpha| \|A\tau - \tilde{b}\|_2 + \lambda^2 |\alpha| \|L\tau\|_2 \tag{5.11}$$

$$= \underset{\tau}{\operatorname{argmin}} \|A\tau - \tilde{b}\|_2 + \lambda^2 \|L\tau\|_2 \tag{5.12}$$

I.e., given that solutions are unique, if τ is the solution to Eq. 5.12, $\alpha\tau$ is the solution to Eq. 5.10, and a scaling error in $\tilde{b}$ would lead to the same scaling error in τ.

Hence, assuming that Δv is not known and considered arbitrary, solutions to Eq. 5.9 may be scaled to match the known range of the true solution, which is the QRS duration [41]:

$$\tau_{T,i} = T \frac{\tau_i - \min_i \tau_i}{\max_i \tau_i - \min_i \tau_i}, \tag{5.13}$$

where T: QRS duration and $i \in 1 \ldots n$ the vector components of τ. Note that the offset correction with $\min_i \tau_i$ in Eq. 5.13 is possible since if τ is a solution to Eq. 5.9, $\tau + \beta,\ \beta \in \mathbb{R}$ is also a solution: in theory, all homogeneous distributions in τ are in the null space of A and L, if A is constructed for transmembrane voltages and L the Laplace operator. Medical doctors in the cath-lab usually refer to the R-peak as LAT $= 0$ ms. To interface with LATs measured in the clinic, τ_R is defined as

$$\tau_R = \tau_T - t_{Rpeak} \tag{5.14}$$

To introduce a set of clinical LAT samples as a priori information the solver is then embedded in a disciplined convex programming [92] framework. To being able to introduce boundary conditions from the measured LATs it is necessary to work in the domain of τ. As a first step, the LATs are converted to τ_T representation:

$$\tau_{Tapr,i} = \begin{cases} \text{LAT}_i + t_{Rpeak} \text{ if LAT of node i available} \\ \text{not defined else} \end{cases} \tag{5.15}$$

Note that LATs are assumed to be measured within the QRS interval and with respect to the R-peak.

Next, conversion to τ is required according to Eq. 5.13. However, as this includes non-linear operations such as min and max, it cannot be done as part of the cost functional. The scaling factor in Eq. 5.13 is instead trained on a previous unconstrained inverse solution with Eq. 5.9:

$$\tau_{T,i} = T \frac{\tau_i - \min_i \tau_i}{\max_i \tau_{Eq.5.9,i} - \min_i \tau_{Eq.5.9,i}} \tag{5.16}$$

$$= \Theta_{Eq.5.9} \left(\tau_i - \min_i \tau_i \right), \tag{5.17}$$

$$\text{where } \Theta_{Eq.5.9} := \frac{T}{\max_i \tau_{Eq.5.9,i} - \min_i \tau_{Eq.5.9,i}} \tag{5.18}$$

To get from τ to τ_T would still require a min operation. However, as noted above for $\tau + \beta$, it is known that an offset in the inverse solution is ineffective in both summands of the cost functional (given the approximation of the Laplace operator has been optimized for this property). Therefore, to impose constraints on τ_T with the intention of finding a better solution τ to the cost functional, the cost functional may as well be computed for $\hat{\tau} = \left(\tau - \min_i \tau_i \right)$, which translates directly back into the original cost functional:

$$A\hat{\tau} = A \left(\tau - \min_i \tau_i \right) = A\tau \tag{5.19}$$

$$L\hat{\tau} = L \left(\tau - \min_i \tau_i \right) = L\tau \tag{5.20}$$

For the purpose of constraining solutions to the cost functional, boundary conditions in τ_T can hence be imposed on τ by a sole correction of scale:

$$\tau_T = \Theta_{Eq.5.9} \tau \tag{5.21}$$

Using the scaling factor from the previous unconstrained solution, the inverse problem is solved in the disciplined convex programming framework of the CVX toolbox for MATLAB [92, 93] with λ from the L-curve of the cost functional in Eq. 5.9 and constraints imposed on the LATs as follows:

$$\tau_{\lambda C} = \underset{\tau}{\operatorname{argmin}} \|A\tau - b\|_2 + \lambda^2 \|L\tau\|_2, \tag{5.22}$$

s.t.

$$\Theta_{Eq.5.9}\tau > lb \tag{5.23}$$

$$\Theta_{Eq.5.9}\tau < ub \tag{5.24}$$

$$\frac{\|\Theta_{Eq.5.9}\tau_S - \tau_{Tapr,S}\|_2}{\sqrt{|S|}} < \eta, \tag{5.25}$$

where $ub = max\left(\left\{\tau_{Tapr,S}, T\right\}\right)$ and $lb = min\left(\left\{\tau_{Tapr,S}, 0\right\}\right)$, $S = \{$ indices where τ_{Tapr} is defined $\}$, $|S|$: cardinality of S such that η: upper bound of the root mean square error in τ_T.
The solution for $\tau_{\lambda C}$ is of course considered to have a wrong offset, due to the imposed constraints and because of Eq. 5.19 and Eq. 5.20, but this does not materialize in the final result: the solution for $\tau_{\lambda C}$ is scaled to the range of τ_T,

$$\tau_{T,\lambda C} = \Theta_{Eq.5.9}\left(\tau_{\lambda C} - min(\tau_{\lambda C})\right), \tag{5.26}$$

and finally converted to activation times with respect to the R-peak:

$$\tau_{R,\lambda C} = \tau_{T,\lambda C} - t_{Rpeak}. \tag{5.27}$$

5.4 Tikhonov Spatio-Temporal Method with BSPM Offset Correction (WIN, OFF, OFFR)

Acknowledging the difficulty of identifying the correct offset in the BSPM, especially for cases of VT[1], an algorithm was proposed to compute an optimized BSPM offset along with the inverse solution. To this end, the inverse problem is solved for a time window, yet evaluated at just a single time point x_{eval}, and the optimal offset is computed for all these time steps together.

$$AX_{\text{window}} = B_{\text{window}}, \tag{5.28}$$

[1] VT baseline correction has been proposed in [94, 95], specifically also for the purpose of ECG imaging. In these works, variations in the heart rate were used to remove T-waves from QRS complexes during VT.

where the time window is represented as

$$X_{\text{window}} = [x_1 \cdots x_T]$$
$$B_{\text{window}} = [b_1 \cdots b_T] \tag{5.29}$$

with T: number of samples in the window.
First, to cope with the dimensionality of an inverse problem with multiple constraints, the time window is reduced to p time vectors using V_p, which contains the first p singular vectors in the temporal basis of the singular value decomposition of B_{window}. The final solution is later transformed back into time space and evaluated at the desired time sample.

$$AX_{\text{window}} = B_{\text{window}} = USV^T \tag{5.30}$$
$$\Leftrightarrow AX_V = BV_p = B_V, \text{ where } V_p \in \mathbb{R}^{T \times p} \tag{5.31}$$

Second, the original problem in Eq. 5.30 is augmented in the solution domain, such that the solution carries additional components $\varepsilon_1, \ldots, \varepsilon_m$ that represent the optimal BSPM offset, i.e. for $b \in \mathbb{R}^{m \times 1}$, m components are added to x and m columns to A:

$$\tilde{x} = \begin{bmatrix} x \\ \varepsilon \end{bmatrix}, \text{ where } x = \begin{bmatrix} x_1 \\ \vdots \\ x_n \end{bmatrix}, \varepsilon = \begin{bmatrix} \varepsilon_1 \\ \vdots \\ \varepsilon_m \end{bmatrix} \tag{5.32}$$

$$\tilde{A} = \left[A \ \text{id.}^{m \times m} \right], A \in \mathbb{R}^{m \times n}, \tag{5.33}$$

such that

$$\tilde{A}x = Ax + \varepsilon = b \tag{5.34}$$

For all temporal singular vectors

$$\tilde{X} = [\tilde{x_1} \dots \tilde{x_p}] \tag{5.35}$$

the following functional is minimized:

$$\begin{aligned} \|A\tilde{X}_V\|_{\text{fro}} + \lambda^2 \|L\tilde{X}_V V_p^T\|_{\text{fro}} \\ \text{s.t.} \\ \varepsilon_1 = \varepsilon_2 = \cdots = \varepsilon_p \\ \varepsilon_i < 0.1,\ i = 1, \dots, m \\ \varepsilon_i > -0.1,\ i = 1, \dots, m \end{aligned} \tag{5.36}$$

From the solution for X_V in $\tilde{X}_V$, the window X_{window} can be computed and the solution can be evaluated at time step x_{eval}:

$$X_{window} = X_V V_p^T \tag{5.37}$$

To provide a reference for the results in Sect. 7.1.4, a variant of the algorithm (WIN) was tested where the augmentation and boundary conditions were dropped. This lead to the following variants of the method:

- WIN: standard Tikhonov spatio-temporal method without offset correction
- OFF: proposed offset correction, time window positioned around the time of evaluation
- OFFR: proposed offset correction, time window positioned around the R-peak

The time window for the WIN scheme and the OFF scheme was positioned around the time of evaluation. For the OFFR scheme, the window was positioned around the R-peak, and the sought x_{eval} was added to the window as the first column. All methods were implemented using the CVX disciplined convex programming framework for MATLAB [92, 93], and they are a variant of Greensite's spatio-temporal Tikhonov approach [96].

5.5 Model-Based Approach

The challenge of the inverse problem of ECG is the underdeterminedness of the solution and the attenuation of its high spatial frequency components in the BSPM. To overcome its difficulties, it is ultimately the goal to introduce as much a-priori knowledge in the solution as possible, while leaving room for its physiological and pathological variations.

It is dangerous to use solely model-based approaches, as they usually do not leave room for these variations unless deviation from the model is permitted, e.g. through stochastic frameworks. Since it can be assumed for the cases in this study that all tissue in the geometric heart model is excitable (except for Patient 12, where scars were identified, see Tab. 7.1), results for the PVC study are also presented for a model-based approach in this work.

While previous works [79–83] have come up with rather advanced data-driven adaptations, e.g. of the excitation conduction velocities, the implementation here follows a simple algorithm that, in contrary e.g. to [79, 81], does not need an initial guess. The proposed method computes the similarities between model-based ECG simulations and the measured ECG, with either the mean temporal (MODcct) or mean spatial correlation coefficient serving as similarity measure (MODccs):

- As in the case of the MAP method, cardiac excitation propagation was modeled as follows: the distance to the excitation origin was computed using the Dijkstra algorithm and weighted with a conduction velocity of 0.8m/s (isotropic, in contrary to that in [79, 81]) to obtain activation times. These were convolved with an action potential template from a simulation with a reaction-diffusion model [97, 98]. Simulations were produced for each 3rd node in the heart mesh to contain the size of the resulting data and forward-calculated with the lead-field matrix.
- The following was repeated for each 3rd node in the heart:
  - Two "agents" were sent out from the R-peak (maximum) of the envelope of the absolute BSPM signal to find the first occurrence of 15% of the R-peak magnitude towards the end and the start of

the beat. This was done for both the measured and the simulated BSPM. The scheme avoids problems with pacing artifacts or ST-segment elevation.

- The identified interval in the simulated BSPM was then interpolated to fit the interval in the measured BSPM, which normalizes for errors in the choice of the conduction velocity.
- Mean temporal or mean spatial correlation coefficients were computed to measure the similarity of the simulation with the measured BSPM.

- The node with the greatest similarity measure was chosen as the excitation origin.

6

Clinical Application - Methods

"There are always inaccuracies in clinical data. In my experience, a method either works without fine-tuning, or it does not work in a clinical context."

Kawal Rhode

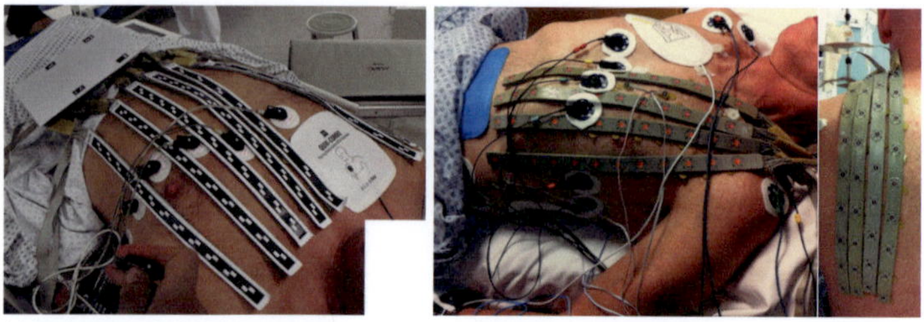

(a) University Medical Center Mannheim (Patient 19).

(b) King's College London (Patient 10).

Figure 6.1: Clinical application of the BioSemi 80-channel BSPM system in the catheter lab. Electrodes were applied on the front of the thorax at University Medical Center Mannheim, where a photogrammetric approach was used for electrode localization. At King's College London a biplane X-ray based localization approach was used, with electrodes on the front and back, but with restrained field of view.

In this chapter, setups and processing pipelines for the ECG imaging application studies will be introduced. Thereby, it shall serve as a methodological documentation of the datasets collected. The scope spans from BSPM and image acquisition to the concurrent recording of intracardiac validation measurements. It further includes the related signal processing and building of computer models of the heart and thorax. Attention has to be given to each step of the modeling and acquisition process, as each one of them by itself is crucial to avoid significant errors in the inverse solutions [38, 99].

6.1 BSPM Acquisition and Setups

BioSemi BSPM System

Electrocardiographic measurements were conducted in the catheter lab using an 80-channel BSPM system by BioSemi B.V., Amsterdam, the Netherlands [100, 101]. Clinical application in the catheter lab is demonstrated in Fig. 6.1 for the setups used in the two cooperating clinics.
The system is particularly well-suited for recording bioelectric signals (active electrodes, amplifiers designed to handle great ranges of common mode signal, driven right leg circuit) and has been used in several previous works of our group [21, 102–105] and other works in ECG

imaging [68]. It competes with mostly equivalent alternatives such as the 3D ECG System by Heartscape Technologies, Inc. [106], which is advertised for as BSPM system for detection of myocardial infarctions [107] — or the Refa system by TMSi B.V., Enschede, the Netherlands, which aims mainly at the electroencephalography (EEG) and electromyography (EMG) market [108, 109]. Both alternative systems are FDA-approved, while the BioSemi system is suited for research applications only.

Electrode Setups and Practical Constraints

While an ideal electrode set-up would sample BSPMs on both the entire front and the back of the patient, practical constraints made it necessary to work with electrodes in only the areas where placement and localization was possible. The studies conducted in this work are particularly difficult in that sense, as they are validation studies that took place in the catheter lab. Electrodes could not be localized in CT scans as e.g. in [59], since the study used MRI to demonstrate ECG imaging as a non-invasive and ßero dosetechnique. Patients could not present for MRI immediately before or after the study for logistical reasons, and the BioSemi active electrodes are not suited for MRI. Therefore, electrodes had to be localized in the catheter lab.
At King's College London, electrodes were hence localized on-site using a newly developed algorithm for biplane X-ray imaging [110, 111], which had to use a narrow field of view to minimize exposure to radiation, but which allowed for localization on both the back and front, see Fig. 6.1(b). With just that narrow field-of-view available, electrodes were therefore only placed on the left half of the thorax surface. At University Medical Center Mannheim the algorithm for biplane X-ray imaging was not available. Instead, a camera-based electrode localization system was developed [112], with much greater field of view, but no ability to localize electrodes on the back, see setup in Fig. 6.1(a).
Furthermore, the resulting setups had to deal with limitations such as the need to give the standard 12-lead ECG and defibrillation patches priority, along with a limited flexibility of the strips which made it necessary to use sub-optimal setups for female patients that leave out

parts of the breast. For female patients, it was identified in a study on realistic setups [26] that it is best to place the electrodes vertically under these circumstances, see Fig.6.2(b). The final setups resulting from such considerations and also from failed localization (not visible) and practical conditions on-site are displayed for each patient in the clinical results, Sect. 7.

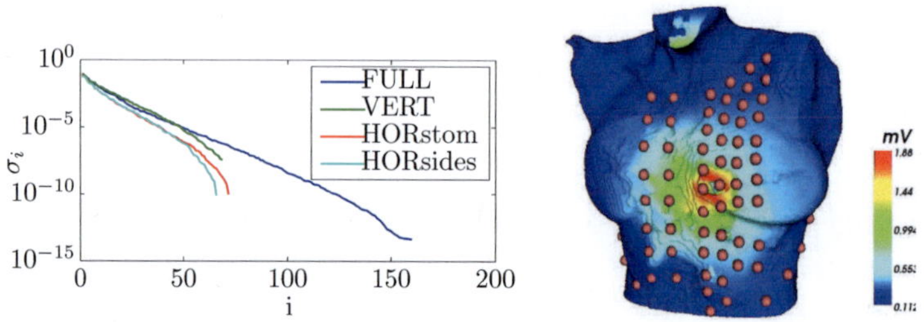

(a) Decay of singular values σ_i in the lead field matrix.

(b) Setup VERT, singular vectors.

Figure 6.2: Different realistic setups for a female patient (Patient 17) were tested for their decay in singular values of the lead field matrix in [26]. (a) FULL: 160 equally distributed electrodes on the front and back, VERT: setup as displayed in (b), HORstom: a horizontal setup with all electrodes below the breasts placed on the stomach, HORsides: horizontal setup with some of these electrodes placed on the sides. (b) The BSPM displayed on the thorax visualizes the sum of the first $i = 1, \cdots, 5$ singular vectors for setup VERT.

6.2 Electrode Localization

For ECG imaging, it is necessary to localize and co-register the electrodes of the BSPM system with great accuracy. While it has been shown that displacement errors of 1 to 2 mm have tolerable impact [113–115], other works have demonstrated that localization errors of 5 mm [38, Sect. 8.1] or 7 mm [116, Sect. 7.3] already impair results significantly. Three electrode localization systems were used in this work:

- a photogrammetric camera-based system (employed at University Medical Center Mannheim) with 1.01 ± 0.51 mm (mean, SD) accuracy, which has been developed and validated within the scope of this work for studies in the catheter lab [112]. The system (Fig. 6.4) facilitates for the first time in ECG imaging a photogrammetry-based electrode localization with automatic marker-based electrode identification. The markers (Fig. 6.1 (a)) are placed on the electrode strips and allow for an identification of BSPM channels with error correction. The code has been published as open source on GitHub [117].

- a biplane X-ray based localization system (King's College London) with 0.33 ± 0.20 mm accuracy as presented in [110]. This system was used for validation measurements in the catheter lab (Fig. 6.3).
- an Optotrak 3020 optical tracking system (King's College London) of sub-millimeter accuracy which is part of the XMR suite at Guy's Hospital, which is presented in [118]. The system was made by Northern Digital Inc., Waterloo, Canada and has previously been used by our group [119]. It was not used for validation studies in the catheter lab, as it is installed in an MRI room. Electrode locations in the XMR suite are recorded with the Optotrak system on the MRI table, and coordinates are produced in the same coordinate system as the MRI data.

The according localization method is referred to in the dataset descriptions in Sect. 7.

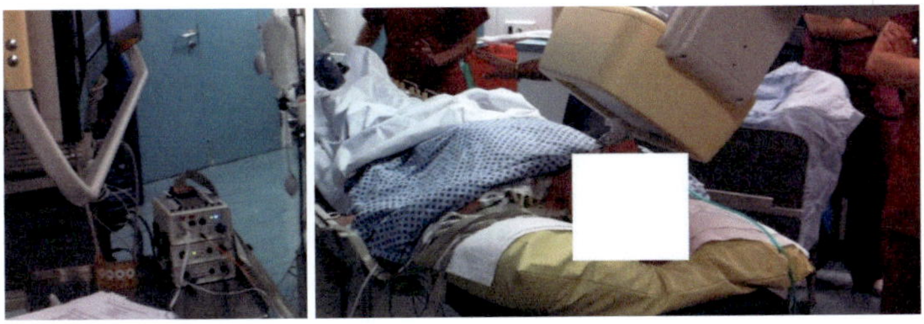

Figure 6.3: Biplane X-ray based electrode localization at King's College London (Patient 10).

6.3 MRI Acquisition and Segmentation Process

3-D anatomical imaging is required to identify tissue structures for computer models of the heart and thorax. While some studies in ECG imaging have used CT [59] and despite CT becoming increasingly efficient, with exposure to radiation decreasing, MRI was used in the studies of this work for its ßero-dosenature. Besides ethical aspects, the non-invasiveness was assumed to be a key requirement for a broad future use of ECG imaging in the clinic. To reduce the logistic efforts of ECGI, fluoroscopy imaging has been proposed as substitute for MRI or CT. It is promising for applications in the catheter lab [121] and may well be combined with the electrode localization method used at King's College [110]. However, the accuracy of fluoroscopy-reconstructed heart geometries with respect to CT-based models was only 10 mm for the human heart in the aforementioned publication (4 mm for a phantom study), which may be considered an unacceptable bias in validation studies as long as ECG imaging is not established with broad empirical evidence of accuracy and robustness. This finding strengthened the decision for MRI.

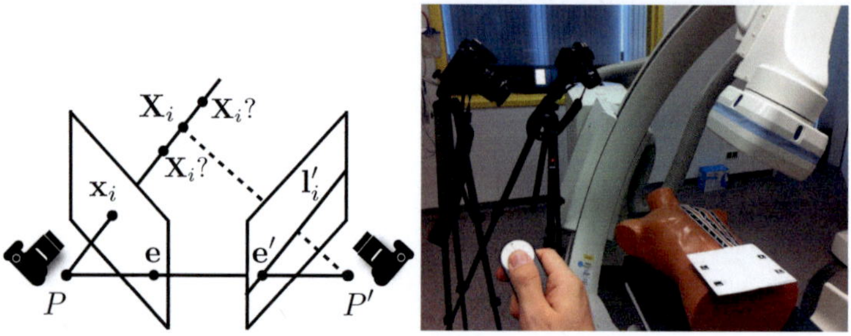

(a) Epipolar geometry used to compute 3-D coordinates from point correspondences in two cameras.

(b) Demonstration in the catheter lab.

Figure 6.4: Setup of the photogrammetric camera-based system that was developed for this project. Fig. (a) is adapted from [120, Fig. 9.1]).

To produce anatomical models of the thorax, imaging of the upper body was required that covered the shoulders (in the sagittal plane), the lateral ends of the body (in the coronal plane) and the back and breasts (in the transversal plane). Heart scans were required to cover the entire ventricles (University Medical Center Mannheim) or the whole heart (King's College London).

Cardiac and respiratory gating issues had to be solved to combine MRI scans of the thorax and heart to form patient geometries. Cardiac images were taken in the end-diastolic phase, which is best suited for ECG imaging of electrical depolarization processes, as the heart is almost at rest during the end-diastolic phase and continues to be so during the QRS complex [122]. Respiratory gating was required as thorax and heart scans as well as acquisitions that are combined to form a heart scan may have different respiratory levels (for an overview of motion artifacts in cardiovascular MR imaging, see [123]). The effect is illustrated in Fig. 6.5(a), where a heart scan is superimposed over a thorax scan. Different schemes were used in the clinical cooperations to handle the gating, as well as the image segmentation.

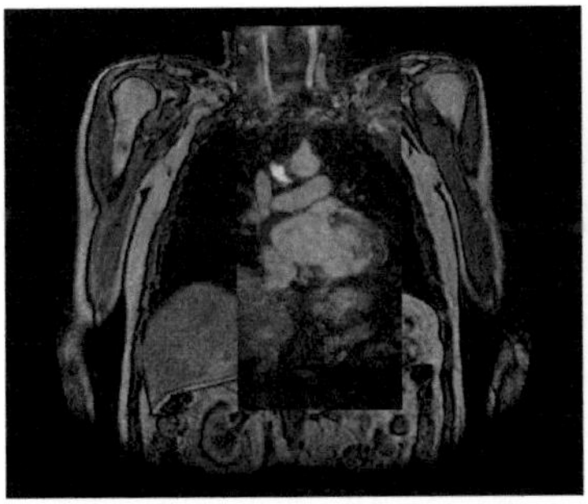

(a) Heart MRI over thorax, Patient 02.

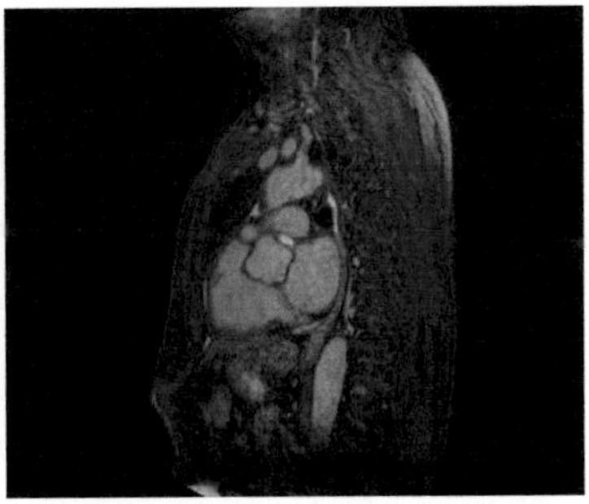

(b) Navigated whole heart MRI, Patient 02.

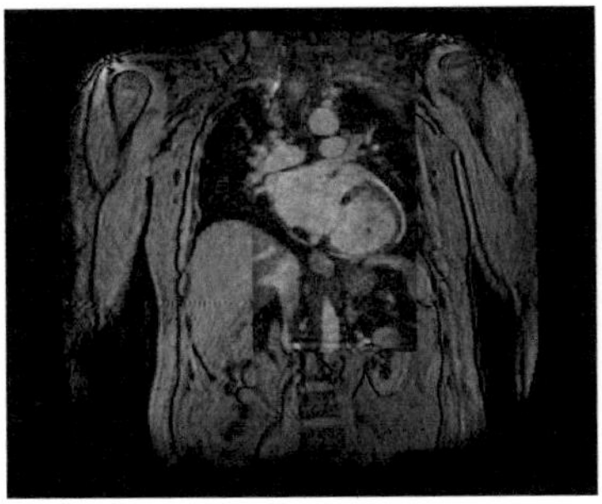

(c) Heart MRI over thorax, Patient 05.

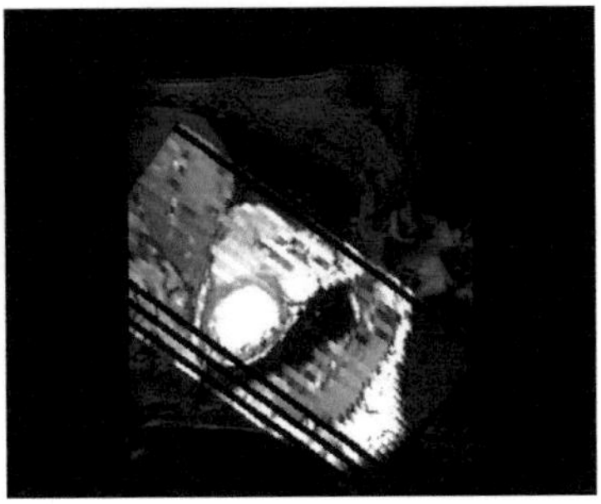

(d) Cine MRI stack over thorax, Patient 20.

Figure 6.5: MRI scans of the thorax and heart, (a)-(c) King's College London, (d) University Medical Center Mannheim.

6.3.1 Imaging at University Medical Center Mannheim

For the clinical study on PVCs, which was conducted in cooperation with University Medical Center Mannheim (UMM), a Siemens 3T

whole-body imaging system [124] (MAGNETOM Skyra, Siemens AG, Healthcare Sector, Erlangen, Germany) with 6-element phased array body coil was used. To obtain images of the thorax a T1-weighted volumetric interpolated breath-hold examination (VIBE) with fat saturation was used, with a 3-D spoiled turbo gradient echo sequence. For the later merger with the heart scan, the VIBE scans that cover the thorax were acquired in multiple breathing levels. Having several scans available, the scan with its respiratory level closest to that of the heart scan could later be selected. Fig. 6.5(d) shows the best match for Patient 20, where a stack of cine MRI images was collected to represent the heart.
To collect standard 3-D whole heart scans navigator triggering [125, 126] was used initially in the study (flash, inversion recovery). Although the method had worked properly with control cases, it provided bad imaging quality for patients with frequent PVCs. Arrhythmia detection, which may be used to exclude arrhythmic beats in the gating, was not used due to the expected considerably extended imaging times and the related stress for the patients. Heart scans were therefore produced from a sequence of cine MRI instead (9 patients). For the patients towards the end of the study, images were picked from one of the following two sequences or the cine MRI, which have the advantage of acquiring the entire heart at once and provide better resolution across slices: an MR-angiography flash-3d scan (Patient 19, resolution: $0.72 \times 0.72\,\mathrm{mm}^2$, slice thickness 1.40 mm) and a T-1 weighted VIBE scan with fat saturation (not chosen for Patient 19 or Patient 20, in which it was applied at a resolution of: $1.74 \times 1.74\,\mathrm{mm}^2$, slice thickness 1.70 mm, using the same sequence as for the thorax images, resolution: between $0.68 \times 0.68\,\mathrm{mm}^2$ and $1.95 \times 1.95\,\mathrm{mm}^2$, slice thickness between 1 mm and 2.2 mm). Both were taken after injection of Gadolinium MRI contrast agent.
In detail, for cine MRI 7-12 short axis views covering the whole left and right ventricle were acquired during repeated end-expiratory breath-holds. These ECG-gated cine images were obtained using a segmented steady-state free-precession sequence (SSFP, parameters: TE / GR 1.2/3.2 ms, temporal resolution 35 ms, in plane spatial resolution $1.4 \times 1.8\,\mathrm{mm}^2$, slice thickness 8 mm, inter-slice gap 2 mm). For segmen-

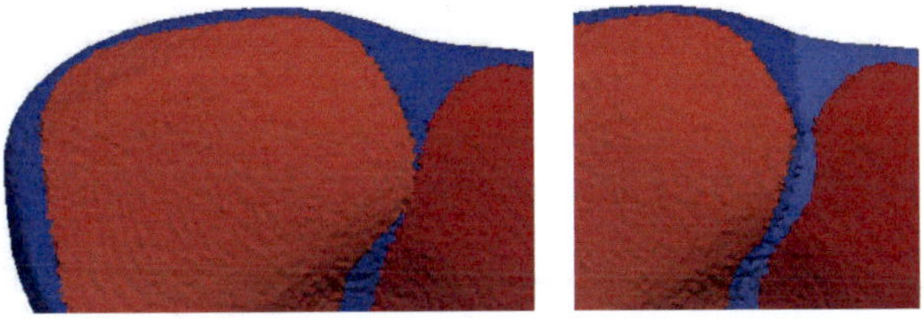

(a) segmentation (b) corrected, RV / LV

Figure 6.6: Segmentation of tissues before (a) and after (b) thickness correction and assignment of RV and LV tissue classes. Red colors: ventricular blood (RV, LV), blue colors: ventricular myocardium (RV, LV), Patient 08.

tation of the ventricles, single images from the end-diastolic phase of each cine sequence were chosen to build a stack of aligned layers (the first images in the cine sequences, which were triggered by the R-peak). Sometimes, these layers were spaced equidistantly to each other, as they resulted from the same collection of short axis views. In some cases, however, data from several such collections was available with the same plane orientation, and information of different collections had to be combined to form the stack. Layers were then extended to the minimum inter-slice distance to their respective neighbours and black spaces were added in the remaining spaces between the layers (see cine MRI stack in Fig. 6.5(d)). Cine MRI has previously been used for heart models in ECG imaging validation studies of ventricular [74] and atrial pre-excitation [68, 76].

For segmentation of the thorax and heart scans, interactively deformable triangle meshes [127] were used in this work on IBT proprietary software. The thorax surface was segmented automatically using foreground masking with Otsu's method as implemented in the brain segmentation plugin of 3D Slicer [128, 129]. The thorax scan was segmented into surface, lungs (left, right), lung vessels (left, right), liver, spleen, stomach, kidney (left, right) and aorta, the heart scan into its ventricular walls and lumina.

After manual segmentation, to prevent models of the heart from having holes, the ventricular walls were tested to have at least a desired minimum thickness, otherwise the segmentation was corrected by growing

the ventricular tissue into the respective blood or non-cardiac tissue (see original segmentation and corrected segmentation of tissues in Fig. 6.6 (a) and Fig. 6.6 (b)). The wall thickness of the RV has been reported in ultrasound studies to be in the order of 3.0 ± 0.92 mm for the diastolic phase and 5.1 ± 1.64 mm in the systolic phase [130], in guidelines it is quantified at 4 mm for the lower reference value estimate in the RV in general and at 2 mm in the RV outflow tract [131][Tab. 2]. The range of reported values according to [132][Tab. 1] also starts at 2 mm. According to [133], LV wall thickness can also be as low as $1-2$ mm in the apex. Still, given the previously mentioned literature values, it was concluded that to perform hole-fixing in the approximate anatomical models built in this study, 2 mm could be set as the appropriate minimum thickness for both the RV and LV.
In the septum, the RV and LV intersect. To distinguish between RV and LV in the segmentation, a rule-based algorithm was used: The geometric distance of cardiac tissue to the respective RV or LV blood was computed. The cardiac tissue closest to the LV blood was assigned the LV tissue class and vice-versa. Due to the distances found in the segmentation of the VISIBLEMAN dataset [134, 135], the wall of the LV was assumed to occupy two thirds of any wall that was found between the two lumina (the blood pools), the RV was assumed to occupy one third of the tissue. For results for the assigned tissue classes see Fig. 6.6 (b).

6.3.2 Imaging at King's College London

For the clinical study on ventricular tachycardia (VT) with King's College London (KCL) the Philips Achieva 1.5T MRI scanner (Philips, Best, The Netherlands) at Guy's Hospital, London, was used. This MRI research suite has the Optotrak electrode localization system installed, see Sect. 6.2. Thorax scans were taken during expiration with a SENSE breath-hold ultra fast gradient echo sequence (resolution: $1.41 \times 1.41\,mm^2$ or $1.48 \times 1.48\,mm^2$, slice thickness 2 mm or 4 mm). An ECG-gated SSFP sequence was then used for MRI acquisitions of the whole heart, including the atria and with high level of detail, see

Fig. 6.5(b). A navigator was used to facilitate respiratory gating (resolutions: $0.87 \times 0.87\,\text{mm}^2$ to $1.21 \times 1.21\,\text{mm}^2$, slice thickness between 0.9 mm and 5 mm). In Patients 05 and 10, proper co-registration of heart and thorax scans was ensured by navigator-triggering at the thorax scan breath-hold level, see Fig. 6.5(c), whereas corrections had to be undertaken manually (which were performed in the axial dimension only) for the other cases, e.g. Patient 02 in Fig. 6.5(a).
Thorax segmentation was performed manually with the PHILIPS CHD segmentation software package provided in the context of the euHeart project (European Community's Seventh Framework Programme) by Philips Research Hamburg, Germany. The tool uses a level set method and allows for a quick, immediately three-dimensional and adaptive generation of segmentations [119]. Heart segmentations were produced automatically with the PHILIPS SSFP cardiac segmentation plug-in [136], which was also provided in the context of the euHeart project by Philips Research. Segmentations of ventricular scar tissue from delayed-enhancement magnetic resonance imaging were provided by King's College London in this study. For details, see [137].

6.3.3 Active Tissue at the Base of the Ventricles

For the segmentations from both studies, it was not possible to differentiate between electrically active tissue at the base of the ventricles and the valves. Hence, the level of the valves is missing in the segmentations. This can be justified, however, as the wall thickness and therefore the signals from this tissue can be assumed to be of negligible strength. For ECG imaging methods that do not work with explicit pathways of excitation conduction (e.g. smoothed TMVs or smoothed activation times) this simplification can be considered to have little effect: although additional active myocardium would result in additional sources and links in the smoothing operators, the absence of tissue does not rule out solutions with pathways through this tissue, and many groups work with that simplification. For methods that require a reconstructed wavefront to travel along a tissue pathway however, especially model-based approaches [80, 81, 138] or fastest-route initial estimates [79], working with the resulting anatomical models may keep such solutions out of the true solution space.

6.4 Mesh Generation and Resolution

To build computer models of the patients for FEM forward calculations, tetrahedral meshes were generated from the aforementioned voxel-based segmentations with tools of the computational geometry algorithms library (CGAL) [139]. A rule-based approach according to Streeter et al. [104, 140] was used to introduce fiber orientation in the ventricles to produce conductivity tensors, with magnitudes set in line with [141]. Meshing parameters were set according to Tab. 6.1. The effect of all relevant parameters on forward-calculated BSPMs had previously been tested in [142] and the appended study in Sect. A. The studies support the proposed setup with the following findings: With the heart tissue refined to 1 mm resolution, only random-noise-related effects were seen in the BSPM upon further refinement. At the same time, the choice is robust, as a lowering of the resolution did not immediately influence the BSPM in [142] and only did so after adding another millimeter in the repetition of the study in Fig. A.2. The facet_angle had little effect and was set to 25° (Fig. A.5). Thorax-related parameters facet_size and cell_size had little impact on the BSPM when the heart was already resolved at 1 mm (Sect. A.2). Both were chosen such that even without refinement of the heart, calculations express similar behaviour as for their highest possible resolution setting, see Fig. A.12 (4 mm and 5 mm). The cell_radius_edge_ratio parameter was not studied and was set to 3 as meshing is guaranteed to converge for it being greater than 2. According to the findings in Sect. A.2, a small facet_distance tends to facilitate a successful meshing procedure. It also prevents the facets from being too far from the surface. Such non-conformal meshes greatly influence electric field calculations [143]. Still, on the other hand, 1 mm was preferred over the most robust setting of 0.5 mm, as to prevent staircase effects from the underlying 0.4 mm voxel-grid with tissue information.

Parameter	Range	Description
		Criteria for surface facets
facet_angle (f_a)	25°	Lower bound for the angles of facets that belong to the surface of the volumetric mesh
facet_size (f_s)	4 mm	Upper bound for the radii of surface Delaunay balls that describe the size of surface facets
facet distance (f_d)	1 mm	Upper bound for the approximation error of boundary and subdivision surfaces of the geometrical pattern
		Criteria for mesh cells
cell_radius_ edge_ratio (c_r_e)	3	Upper bound for the circumradius-to-shortest-edge ratio
cell_size (c_s)	5 mm	Upper bound for the circumradius
		Criteria for refined tissues
refine_facet_size (r_f_s)	same as facet_size	(heart tissue)
refine_cell_size (r_c_s)	1 mm	(heart tissue)

Table 6.1: Proposed setup for CGAL mesh generation parameters. For more information on the parameters, see [142].

To represent sources of TMVs in the forward calculations a coarse mesh of 4 mm resolution was used. Lead field matrices were produced with the bidomain model (Sect. 3.2). The TMVs from the coarse mesh were interpolated for this purpose on the fine mesh of the heart.

For calculations with the boundary element method (BEM) the surface of the FEM thorax meshes and coarse heart meshes were extracted, simplified (vertex simplification with quadric edge collapse decimation) and smoothed in MeshLab [144], which is a tool developed with the support of the 3D-CoForm project. Smoothing was performed on the face normals using a method that preserves the positions of the vertices and prevents the models from shrinking. Models for BEM contain only the thorax and heart surfaces, with isotropic conductivities assigned to the heart ($0.1\,S/m$) and thorax ($0.2\,S/m$). For surface TMV calculations also the intracellular space of the myocardium ($0.05\,S/m$) was considered.

6.5 Rigid Co-Registration of Electrodes with the Thorax Model

At UMM, after localization (Sect. 6.2), electrode positions of the 80-channel body surface potential mapping (BSPM) system were rigidly co-registered with the thorax model using anatomical landmarks such as nipples, liver spots, intersections of prominent veins, prominent bone structures or tattoos. These landmarks were either also visible in the MRI or marked with MRI-compatible electrodes. Co-registration was performed numerically, but with the landmarks weighted according to their assumed reliability, which was judged mostly by the volume coverage and visibility of the respective fiducial in the MRI (documented in the datasets). To identify a rigid transformation between the corresponding landmarks, the underlying 3-D point co-registration (introduced here without the weighting) was performed as follows:

According to a scheme presented in [145, 146], to identify the optimal rotation and translation between corresponding 3D points $p_A^i \in \mathbb{R}^{3\times 1}$ and $p_B^i \in \mathbb{R}^{3\times 1}$,

$$Rp_A^i + t = p_B^i, \; i = 1 \cdots N, \tag{6.1}$$

both a translation $t \in \mathbb{R}^{3\times 1}$ and a rotation matrix $R \in \mathbb{R}^{3\times 3}$ were produced such that

$$\min_{R,t} \sum_{i=1}^{N} \|Rp_A^i + t - p_B^i\|.$$

To this end, the covariance of the point data was computed and decomposed into its singular values. A matrix $\tilde{R}$ was then derived from the resulting bases:

$$\begin{aligned} C = \frac{1}{N}\sum_{i=1}^{N}\left(p_A^i - \frac{1}{N}\sum_{i=1}^{N} p_A^i\right)\left(p_B^i - \frac{1}{N}\sum_{i=1}^{N} p_B^i\right)^T \\ USV^T = \mathrm{svd}(C) \\ \tilde{R} = VU^T \end{aligned} \tag{6.2}$$

$\tilde{R}$ may be a rotation matrix or a reflection matrix. To ensure a rotation is obtained the latter case was corrected for by manipulation of V:

$$R = \begin{cases} \begin{pmatrix} v_1, v_2, -v_3 \end{pmatrix} U^T & \text{if } \det \tilde{R} < 0 \\ \tilde{R} & \text{else} \end{cases}, \quad V = \begin{pmatrix} v_1, v_2, v_3 \end{pmatrix} \tag{6.3}$$

The translation was then computed as

$$t = \left(\frac{1}{N} \sum_{i=1}^{N} p_B^i \right) - R \left(\frac{1}{N} \sum_{i=1}^{N} p_A^i \right) \tag{6.4}$$

Note that to guarantee the final transformation does not include a scaling and is indeed rigid, R had to comply with the following criterion of equivalence for rotation matrices [147]:

$$R^{-1} = R^T$$
$$\det R = 1$$

This is guaranteed by the above algorithm, as orthogonality is already guaranteed for the bases of the SVD and therefore also for their transposes and product in Eq. 6.2. The determinant may then be -1 or $+1$, with the latter being guaranteed by the correction in Eq. 6.3.
At KCL, electrodes were localized using the biplane X-ray imaging system (Fig. 6.1). Co-registration with the MRI-based thorax surface was performed using rigid body registration for four electrode markers that appeared in both MRI and X-ray.

6.6 BSPM Processing and Filtering

This section documents the overall handling of electrode channels in the BSPM and the lead field matrix, including the proper choice of reference electrodes, choice of BSPM channels and the filtering.

6.6.1 Choice of a Reference Electrode

After co-registration of the electrodes with the thorax, a reference electrode had to be chosen. Signals in the Biosemi system were recorded with a driven-right-leg circuit: to prevent the recorded signal from going beyond the amplifiers' input voltage range, common mode voltage is actively reduced [148]. To this end, a common mode signal (CMS) was sampled from close to the body center. All 80 channels were recorded with respect to a ground electrode (DRL), which was placed close to the hips or on the waist.
For the forward model that was used to produce the lead field matrix, which again was later on used to solve the inverse problem, a zero potential had to be defined as well, which had to comply with the zero potential definition in the given BSPM.
As the position of the DRL reference electrode had not been reproduced with the localization system[1], a new reference had to be defined among the recorded channels. The method of choosing the reference is outlined in the following, and it is highlighted that a good reference has impact on the inverse solution.

Effect on the Inverse Solution

As all electrode signals are processed with respect to the reference, noise on the reference channel is added to all other channels, leading to its representation in all elements of the measurement vector b in the inverse problem. I.e., assuming absence of other errors, if the residual is represented in the inverse calculations with L1 norm, any error in the reference channel will be represented $m-1$ times in the cost (m electrodes), which imposes more bias on the cost than its representation in the single channel. The effect is similar for L2 norm residuals.

Criteria for Choosing a Reference Electrode

From the arguments in the previous paragraph, the most obvious choice for a reference would be the channel with the least assumed noise. An

[1] CMS and DRL electrodes were not provided markers in the camera-based localization system. Also, multiple DRL leads were placed and often switched during the measurement depending on signal quality, which made a post-measurement assignment difficult.

ideal channel would have the least assumed error with respect to the signal generated by the cardiac electric activity (e.g., the least standard deviation over time, assuming it relates to noise and baseline wander). While this minimizes the error that is introduced by the reference channel on all other channels, another approach is more effective: to find a reference that contains the common signal and that therefore compensates as much noise as possible in all of the channels. This is proposed in [149], where Wilson's central terminal is used as the reference in ECG imaging. Here, instead of sticking with Wilson's definition, the average of all signals in the BSPM was computed. As a side-effect, using the average signal as reference saves the electrode channel that is otherwise used as ground. Still, the costöf the averaging on the other hand is loosing effectively the information of 1 of 80 channels.

A Reference which Contains the Common Signal (CN)

The choice of the average over all signals as reference leads to a linear combination of signals, which cannot be implemented as Dirichlet boundary condition in the present FEM-based tools at IBT (an approach is suggested in [149]). Instead, the reference was introduced after having already computed the lead field matrix A (with an arbitrary extra electrode position as ground). This results in A_{CNREF}, which is sought in the following as the mapping from TMVs x to the BSPM with common signal reference b_{CNREF}, which is defined as:

$$A(x - x_{\mathrm{mean}}) = b - b_{\mathrm{mean}} := b_{\mathrm{CNREF}}. \tag{6.5}$$

x_{mean} is the source that would produce $Ax_{\mathrm{mean}} = b_{\mathrm{mean}}$. This shall be the average over all signals in the BSPM:

$$b_{\mathrm{mean}} := \left(\sum_{j=1}^{m} \frac{b_j}{m} \right) \mathbb{1}^{m \times 1},\ b \in \mathbb{R}^{m \times 1} \tag{6.6}$$

With Eq. 4.5, Eq. 6.5 can be written as

$$[\hat{a}_1, \hat{a}_2, \ldots, \hat{a}_n]\,(x - x_{\mathrm{mean}}) = A(x - x_{\mathrm{mean}}) = b_{\mathrm{CNREF}}.$$

To solve the inverse problem for x, not $(x - x_{\text{mean}})$, it would be useful to integrate the subtraction of x_{mean} into a modified lead field matrix A_{CNREF} which would produce b_{CNREF} immediately from x. The following formula is proposed:

$$A_{\text{CNREF}}x := [(\hat{a}_1 - \hat{a}_{1,\text{mean}}), (\hat{a}_2 - \hat{a}_{2,\text{mean}}), \dots \\ , (\hat{a}_n - \hat{a}_{n,\text{mean}})]\, x = b_{\text{CNREF}}, \tag{6.7}$$

$$\hat{a}_{i,\text{mean}} := \left(\sum_{j=1}^{m} \frac{\hat{a}_{i,j}}{m} \right) \mathbb{1}^{m\times 1}, \; \hat{a}_i \in \mathbb{R}^{m\times 1}. \tag{6.8}$$

For Eq. 6.8 to actually produce b_{CNREF}, it must be proven that

$$[\hat{a}_1, \hat{a}_2, \dots, \hat{a}_n]\, x - [\hat{a}_{1,\text{mean}}, \hat{a}_{2,\text{mean}}, \dots, \hat{a}_{n,\text{mean}}]\, x = b - b_{\text{mean}},$$

which is indeed the case:

$$\overset{Eq.\ 4.5}{\Leftrightarrow} [\hat{a}_{1,\text{mean}}, \hat{a}_{2,\text{mean}}, \dots, \hat{a}_{n,\text{mean}}]\, x = b_{\text{mean}}$$

$$\Leftrightarrow \mathbb{1}^{m\times 1} \left(\sum_{j=1}^{m} \frac{\hat{a}_{1,j}x_1 + \hat{a}_{2,j}x_2 + \dots + \hat{a}_{n,j}x_n}{m} \right) = \mathbb{1}^{m\times 1} \left(\sum_{j=1}^{m} \frac{b_j}{m} \right)$$

q.e.d.

The inverse problem can now be solved for

$$A_{\text{CNREF}}x = b_{\text{CNREF}}, \tag{6.9}$$

where the reference in the BSPM is the common signal of all BSPM channels. Note that to compute A_{CNREF} according to Eq. 6.8, one simply subtracts the average from each column in the original lead field matrix A.

6.6.2 Choice of Electrode Signals and Handling of Channels

Among the available channels, electrode signals were excluded from inverse calculations in case of strong signal offsets (great mean over time), which were interpreted as a result of bad electrode contact. Also, outliers in the standard deviation over time were excluded. Both the

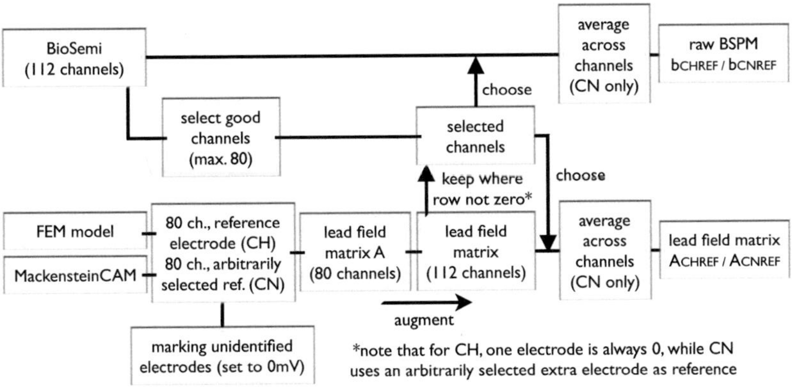

Figure 6.7: BSPM processing flow chart: selection of channels and reference definition.

signals of outliers and those of the selected channels were again plotted over time as visual cross-check. The respective channels had to be handled consistently across the processing of BSPM signals and the computation of lead field matrices, see Fig. 6.7. Besides a censoring of BSPM channels, it was also required to handle missing channels in the electrode localization. Unidentified channels in the localization were therefore set to zero in the lead field matrix calculation (ünidentified electrodesïn Fig. 6.7) and cancelled from the list of ßelected channelsïn the BSPM. Finally, these selected channels were chosen from both the computed lead field matrix and the BSPM, which went into the signal filtering (Fig. 6.8) as "raw BSPM".

6.6.3 Annotation and Filtering

For the UMM study with its PVCs and pacings, beats in the BSPM signals were segmented with annotations at the onset of the QRS or at the last sampling before the pacing (for paced beats) — and at the end of the QRS. As PVCs have long QRS durations, they sometimes overlap with the T-wave. In these cases the end-of-QRS mark was set to the end of the strongest QRS-slope. BSPM signals were then processed as illustrated in Fig. 6.8: BSPMs were acquired at 2048 Hz, resampled with 1000 Hz and then filtered using a 50 Hz notch filter (bandwidth 0.2 Hz). For the subsequent filters to start without oscillations, the average signal between −20 ms and the QRS onset was then removed for each individual channel, assuming that the interval accommodated no cardiac electric activity. After that, a Gaussian low-pass filter with 400 Hz cutoff frequency was applied, and subsequently a Gaussian high-pass filter with 0.3 Hz cutoff frequency. The passband cutoff frequencies were chosen as in the works of Tilg et al. [68, 150].

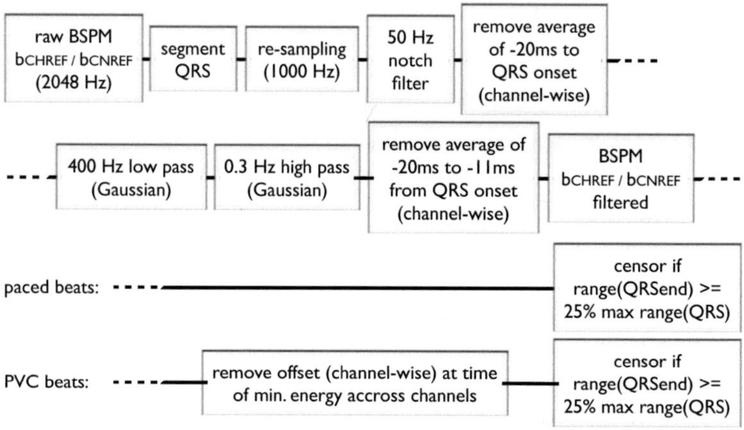

Figure 6.8: BSPM processing flow chart: signal filtering

To obtain only the signal components that can be generated by cardiac electric activity it was crucial to eliminate offsets in the BSPM signals. While high-pass filtering eliminates the signal average in time, it does not necessarily cancel the offset at the beginning of a cardiac event. Therefore, in addition to removing the baseline wander, which is taken care of by the filters, the filtered signals needed further processing to correct the baseline offset.

Following the filtering, under the assumption of absent cardiac electric activity, the average signal between −20 ms and −11 ms with respect to the QRS onset was removed from each individual channel (see Fig. 6.9 (a)). This step was effectively only applied for paced beats. For PVC beats, any remaining offset on the channels was removed instead as follows (see Fig. 6.9(b,c)): Between 1 and 52 ms the signal energy across all channels was summarized for a moving window covering the 8 ms after each time step. The signal of the time step with least energy was thereupon taken as the reference. I.e., practically, all channels at this time start at 0 mV. In contrary to the paced beats, PVCs could be assumed to start where no cardiac activity was present, which was hypothesized to be represented in the signal energy.

Finally, as beats with strong baseline wander (see Fig. 6.10, compared to Fig. 6.9) were presumed to be linked to stronger artifacts in ECG imaging and greater localization error, beats were censored and not considered in the study when the BSPM range at the QRS end was larger than a quarter of its maximum range. Besides baseline wander, this scheme also censors beats when single BSPM channels disconnect during the experiment, i.e. if they start to carry strong noise that had not been detected during the outlier detection phase.

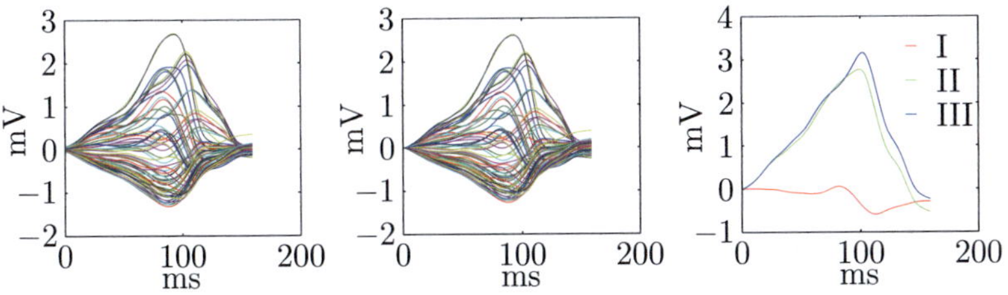

(a) 0 mV: average before onset. (b) 0 mV: min. $\|\mathrm{BSPM}_{8\,\mathrm{ms}}\|_2^2$. (c) Standard leads in (b).

Figure 6.9: Effect of offset removal: Patient 20, PVC beat 1 (early in the dataset, not censored).

For the VT study at KCL, the same filtering schemes were applied. However, as VT beats appear in a long sequence of uninterrupted activity, the QRS onset and offset could not be used for offset removal or beat censoring. Instead, to remove relative offsets between the signals, which are usually significant, spatial smoothness was imposed on the signals at their respective electrode positions, and the average from each electrode channel was removed at the same time by minimizing the following optimization functional:

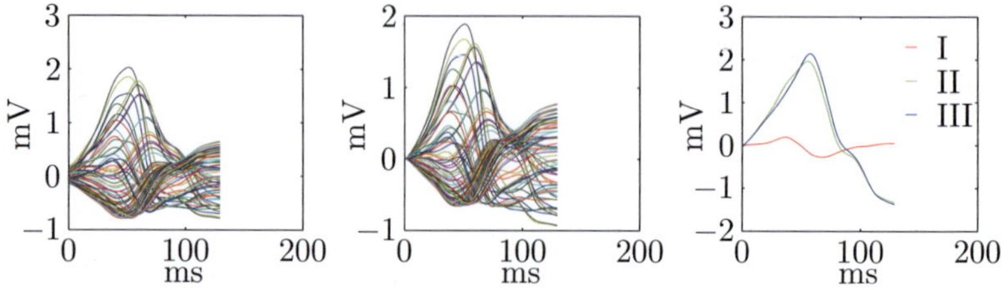

(a) 0 mV: average before onset. (b) 0 mV: min. $||\text{BSPM}_{8\,\text{ms}}||_2^2$. (c) Standard leads in (b).

Figure 6.10: Effect of offset removal: Patient 20, PVC beat 4 (half an hour into the dataset, beat censored).

$$\min_{b_r} ||(B - B_r)||_{fro} + ||G(B - B_r)||_{fro}, \tag{6.10}$$

$$B = [b(t = 1), \ldots, b(t = T)] \tag{6.11}$$

$$B_r = [b_r, \ldots, b_r] \tag{6.12}$$

where b_r is the sought reference signal to be deduced from the BSPM signal $b(t), t = 1 \ldots T$ is the annotated time interval of the cardiac event (VT sequence) and G is a smoothing matrix which computes the spatial gradient between electrode signals.

Note again that removing the average alone, which is also the effect of high-pass filtering in the Fourier domain, eliminates the signal average in time, but does not necessarily cancel the offset at the beginning of the cardiac event.

6.7 Validation Measurements

For validation measurements, the BioSemi BSPM system was applied in the catheter lab while the patient was undergoing an RF ablation procedure. While in [68] radiotransparent carbon electrodes and carbon cables had been used to avoid interference with the biplane X-ray system [68][Sect. II, A.], the electrodes used in this study were made from a powder of silver (Ag) and silver-chloride (AgCl), which is clearly visible in the X-ray images [110, 151]. X-ray was only applied to control substantial active movements of the intracardiac electrode catheters, see

Fig. 6.11. Fine adjustments have been performed with the 3-D-mapping system. While procedures at UMM and KCL were partially guided by X-ray (and partially by an electroanatomical mapping system), cardiologists of the clinical partners found that the setup did not obstruct relevant fields of view during the procedures and did not increase the radiation exposure for the patient. The Ag-AgCl electrodes used in this study were connected with X-ray invisible carbon cables as in [68]. At the same time, they have the benefit of a better signal quality compared to carbon electrodes, which suffer from much larger low-frequency noise.

For the validation study at UMM (Sect. 6.7.1 and 6.7.2), concurrent electroanatomical contact mapping with CARTO® of Biosense Webster, Inc., was performed [152, 153], with single-point catheter measurements directly on the wall serving as validation reference. This has been the standard for validation in ECG imaging since electroanatomical mapping has become available [71]. For the validation study at KCL (Sect. 6.7.3), activation maps of ventricular tachycardia were recorded while measuring BSPMs, which is an event that cannot be repeatedly measured. To being able to map the cardiac electric activity at once, non-contact multichannel mapping had to be used [154, 155]. Instead of performing direct measurements, the EnSite system [156–158] of St. Jude Medical, Inc., was used, which computes activation maps from balloon catheter measurements for a simplified model of the endocardium.

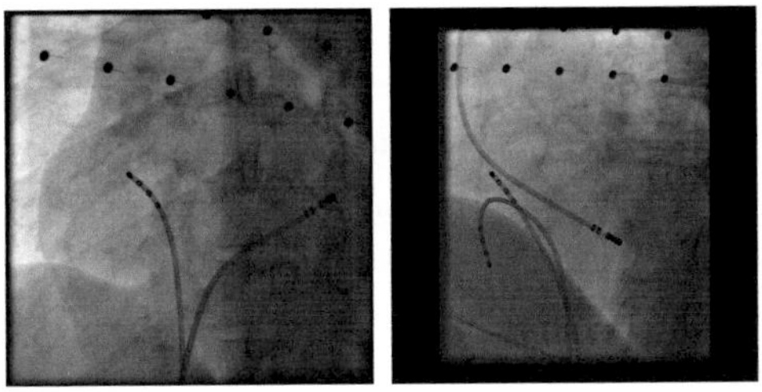

(a) Patient 06, zoom: 194%. (b) Patient 09, zoom: 97%.

Figure 6.11: X-ray images (angle: 0°) showing catheters and the active electrodes of the BioSemi system.

6.7.1 Post-Processing of CARTO Electroanatomical Maps

At UMM, local activation time (LAT) measurements of PVCs and pacing locations were collected using electroanatomical contact mapping with CARTO. The annotations performed in the clinic needed further classification, as measurement points were also collected from cardiac events other than the PVC (e.g. pacing sites or anatomical landmarks with His signal, with distinct purposes in the co-registration or validation procedure). Also, not all measurements and location tags in the CARTO electroanatomical maps were equally reliable. To ensure a good quality of the map used for validation of the ECG imaging study, samplings that were not suitable for creating an LAT map of the PVC were censored and neglected in the map creation, according to the following guideline:

- ablation points were excluded, see Fig. 6.12(g)
- stimulation points were excluded, Fig. 6.12(f)
- beats of different morphology than the sought PVC were excluded (including normal sinus rhythm, NSR), see Fig. 6.12(e)
- the remaining points were judged by the quality of the electrograms. Noisy measurements were excluded, see Fig. 6.12(d), measurements with good signal quality were selected for the activation time map, see Fig. 6.12(a) and Fig. 6.12(b). Annotations were adjusted in case they had been neglected for the map in the clinical procedure, see Fig. 6.12(c).

Note that the best practice to annotate electrograms for LAT mapping is subject to research, and variations in this validation ground truth are possible, depending on the operator and methodology. As an alternative to the bipolar signals used, unipolar electrograms have been demonstrated to show more stable characteristics with respect to the activation time, also under different catheter angles [159]. However, they are also subject to far-field signals and noise. To handle the downsides of both signal types, recent works have suggested algorithms that first find time windows of bipolar activity and that finally annotate the LATs based on characteristics in the unipolar signal within that window [160].

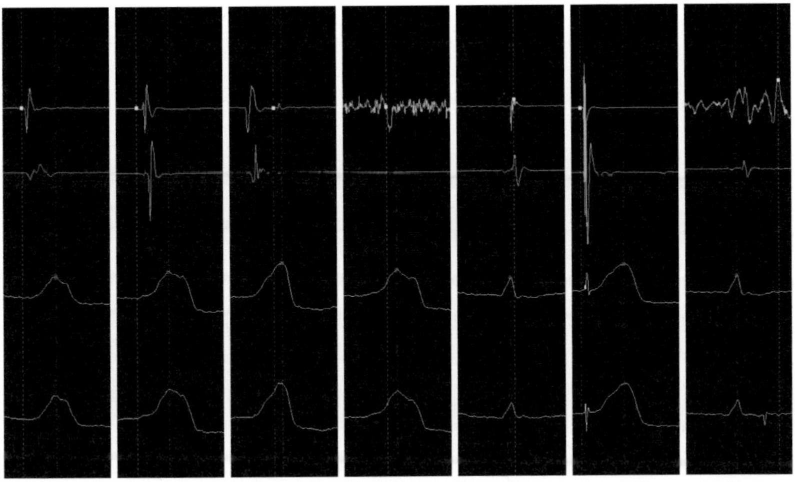

(a) PVC (b) PVC (c) PVC, adjust (d) PVC, noisy (e) not the PVC (f) paced beat (g) ablation

Figure 6.12: Electrograms measured with the CARTO system (top row to bottom row: MAP 1-2, MAP 3-4, V4, Wilson III) and annotations for local activation times (LATs) in the heart (yellow) with respect to the R-peak (red).

In this work, no automatic annotation was used, and decisions were made by the clinical operator.

6.7.2 Co-Registration of CARTO Maps with the MRI-Based Model

An iterative closest point (ICP) algorithm [161] was used to co-register the CARTO LAT maps with the MRI-based heart model. The ICP algorithm has been used for co-registration of electroanatomical maps in [162] and is typically the method-of-choice. Still, ICP algorithms may fail in some cases if the co-registered surfaces are too different in shape, and landmark-based approaches may be preferred for such cases [163]. In this work, to detect such failure, results were tested by visual inspection. Also, the quality of co-registration was quantitatively evaluated by computing the distance of the co-registered points to the endocardial surface, see Sect. 7. In ECGI validation studies by Seger et al. [48] landmark points were collected with the electroanatomical mapping system (EAMS) among the same fiducial markers that were used for

BSPM-electrodes-to-model co-registration. In this study, co-registration is performed directly to the heart to avoid errors from the alignment of the heart MRI with the model of the thorax.
An ICP algorithm was implemented using the algorithm by Wilm and Kjer [164, 165]. The approach was adapted to handle multiple point sets and corresponding reference point sets simultaneously. A weighting of the individual point clouds was introduced to balance their influence in the final co-registration. Registered entities were in particular:

- the lumen/ lumina of the respective ventricle(s)
  (As reference for all points in the respective CARTO map, vertices were used from a triangulation of the MRI-based heart model with 1 mm cell size.)
- the endocardial surface of the respective ventricle(s)
  (Extracted from the aforementioned triangulation, as second reference to register all points in the CARTO map.)

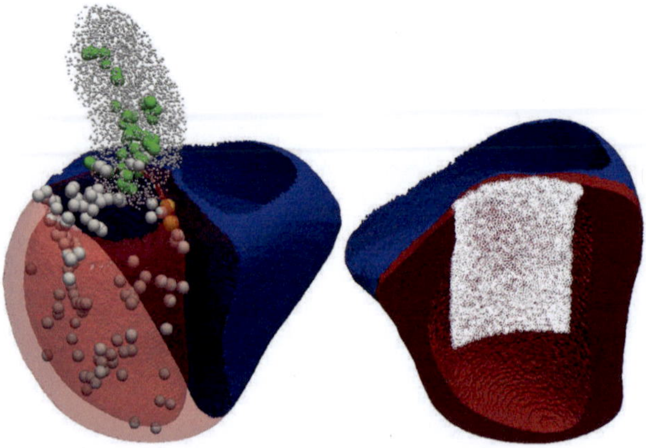

(a) Co-Reg (b) HIS, lateral view

Figure 6.13: Co-registration of CARTO data with MRI-based heart and vessel models, Patient 20. (a) Co-Reg: co-registration of CARTO measurement points (grey), vessel tag points of the aorta (green) and points with HIS signal (yellow) to the MRI-based heart model with the implemented ICP algorithm (weighting LV volume : LV surface : LV His region : vessel tag aorta was 1:10:1:3). A navigated-MRI-based segmentation of the aorta (grey dots) is used as a reference for the vessel tag. (b) HIS: Regions of interest (ROI) for area of possible measurements from the bundle of His.

- the septal surface of the respective ventricle(s) close to the bundle of His
  (Used to register measurement points with bundle-of-His signal [166][Fig. 2].) As reference, the area of possible measurements for signals from the bundle of His was selected from the MRI-based heart model — under the following considerations: the right and left bundle branches belong to the bundle of His and may produce similar signals as the trunk of the bundle; the entire bundle is located in the interventricular septum [167]; it originates at the AV node and descends down into bundle branches in the apex [168][Fig. 501]; in anterior-inferior dimension, the branches may spread immediately at the base from the center to the sides [167][Fig. 12]; hence signals from the bundle of His may be measured in the entire septum. However, annotations in the clinic were only made in case of great H-S intervals between the His bundle spike (H) and the S wave of the ECG, and signals must therefore originate from the upper two-thirds of the septum, which was therefore finally chosen as the registration reference. An example for a segmented reference point cloud is shown in Fig. 6.13.
- segmentations of the clinically annotated vessels
  (To produce vessel tags, the path of the catheter was recorded while retracting from the respective vessel. A corresponding reference was obtained by segmentation of the vessel in the MRI data, see Fig. 6.13)

The result of a co-registration process with three differently weighted point clouds is shown in Fig. 6.13. After co-registration, the closest points of the CARTO LAT measurements were located in the coarse heart mesh in which the inverse problem was solved. In case multiple measurements were taken from the vicinity of the same node in the coarse mesh, LATs were averaged, leading to a mean and standard deviation of measured LATs at the point. This method leads to a very sparse representation of data, but represented the reality of having only few PVC beats available for mapping during a cardiac intervention - and it avoids interpolation or extrapolation. The assigned LATs in the coarse cardiac geometry for Patient 20, including their standard deviation, are shown in Fig. B.9.

6.7.3 EnSite Non-Contact Maps

For the VT study at KCL, non-contact mapping with the EnSite system was performed, with a balloon catheter placed in the LV while measuring the BSPM. This system produces a shell model of the LV, which was registered with the MRI-based LV model using anatomical landmark registration. The results of this co-registration are documented in [137, Fig. 1 (a),(b)].

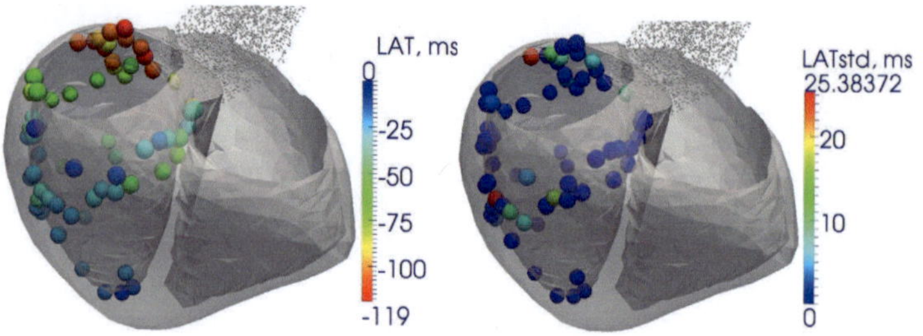

(a) Patient 20, LAT (b) Patient 20, std(LAT)

Figure 6.14: Assignment of LAT measurements to the coarse cardiac geometry. Multiple assignments to the same position are averaged (a), with the standard deviation displayed in (b).

Part III

Results

7

Clinical Studies

"We have done the talking and we now need to see the results in action."

Jan Egeland

With the methods from the previous chapter it was possible to apply ECG imaging in a clinical environment. This work has focused on two clinical validation studies, which were intended to demonstrate how ECG imaging methods work in humans. Through cooperation with the University Medical Center Mannheim (UMM) and with King's College London (KCL) it was possible to perform studies with intracardiac validation measurements that were collected in the ventricles while measuring the BSPM at the same time. The study with UMM includes PVCs as well as pacings from various known positions and local activation time maps of the PVCs that were obtained with a contact mapping system. This facilitates two things: the validation of ECG imaging in terms of localizing excitation origins and the validation of its ability to image activation times. The study at KCL captured the cardiac electric activity of a sustained VT. Happening only once in a study, to produce a map of local activation times the VT was recorded with a non-contact mapping system with a balloon catheter inserted in the left ventricle. While ECG imaging is non-invasive, invasive measurements are needed to facilitate its validation. All clinical studies in this work were approved by the local ethics committees, and written informed consent was obtained from the patients.

7.1 Validation Study: Premature Ventricular Contractions

Electroanatomical maps of PVCs were recorded during radiofrequency ablation therapies in the Stereotaxis lab [169] at UMM. Measurements include local activation time maps, pacing positions as well as ablation points that were collected with the CARTO contact mapping system while measuring the BSPM at the same time. The study includes 8 patients with a complete set of validation measurements, see Tab. 7.1. Patient 06 has only a very incomplete electroanatomical map, but is evaluated here as well. Patient 08 has a complete model, but intracardiac measurements could not be studied due to cancellation of the study. The following patient datasets were excluded from presentation: Patient 04 (MRI, BSPM and biplane X-ray catheter images are available, evaluation was cancelled due to incomplete MRI scans), Patient 07 (BSPM available,

no catheterization due to lack of arrhythmic activity, did not show up for MRI), Patients 15 and 16 (MRI test cases), Patient 18 (test case for MRI protocols, BSPM, no validation data).
Datasets for ECG imaging are a complex fusion of multiple imaging and measurement modalities that have to be co-registered, and only in case of good data collection and registration in each single one of these steps the resulting models can be assumed to represent the patient's anatomy and electrophysiology. While the upper block in Tab. 7.1 characterizes the type and quality of the recorded excitation origins (distance to the heart mesh used for ECG imaging), the lower sections give an overview of the modeling steps and their quality, according to quantitative or otherwise non-quantitative objective criteria (for details, see B in the Appendix).

Patient-ID	6	8	9	11	12	13	14	17	19	20
Myocardial infarction	0	0	0	0	1	0	0	0	0	0
Ablation therapy successful	C	C	1	?	0	1	C	1	1	1
Annotated excitation origin	ET	C	ET	ET	ET	MA	ET	ET	ET	ET
distance coarse mesh BEM [mm]	6	C	8	6	8	7	7	8	6	13
distance coarse mesh FEM [mm]	2	C	6	3	8	6	1	6	4	13
Segmentation thorax organs	++	++	++	++	++	++	++	++	++	++
Segmentation thorax surface	+	+	++	++	++	++	++	+	++	++
Segmentation heart	++	++	+	x	+	++	++	++	+	++
Co-registration heart and thorax	++	+	+	x	+	+	++	+	++	++
Electrode localization	+	+	+	++	x	++	++	++	++	++
Electrode co-registration	x	x	x	x	x	x	++	+	+	++
CARTO activation times	x	C	+	++	++	+	++	+	++	++
CARTO anatomical map	x	C	++	+	++	+	++	+	++	++
CARTO co-registration	+	C	+	++	+	++	++	++	++	++
BSPM of pacings	0	0	1	1	1	1	1	1	1	1

Table 7.1: List of Patients. Quality of features evaluated by quantitative or otherwise non-quantitative objective criteria (see Tables in Sect. B.2). Legend: x sufficient quality achieved (partially through manual efforts), + OK quality, ++ good quality, C not available/ therapy cancelled (no ablations), ? significantly reduced frequency of PVCs during therapy, ET: point of earliest reliably measured activation time is used as validation reference for excitation origins of the PVC, MA: mean position of ablation points, as latest successful ablation unknown and activation times only available for QRS.

7.1.1 Presentation of Results

As a proof-of-concept, convincing and nice-looking ECG imaging results can easily be obtained when presenting best-cases with ideally parameterized solvers. E.g., the imaging of transmembrane voltages of single time points can nicely be shown to lead to successful localization of the PVC origin, see Fig. 7.1, looking more accurate even than the validation measurements (PVC origins: bullets in magenta [1]). However, in this work, it shall be acknowledged that it is difficult to optimize the regularization parameters, given that many possible choices exist that so far cannot be distinguished from the non-invasive clinical data alone (see [170] for a potential solution to this problem). Results in the subsequent sections are hence presented with either a fix parameterization used across the patient population or with the regularization parameters chosen according to automatic schemes. Further, results in Fig. 7.1 are presented for just a single beat of the PVC, while it shall be shown in this work whether results are robust over a sequence of beats that originate from the same cardiac event.

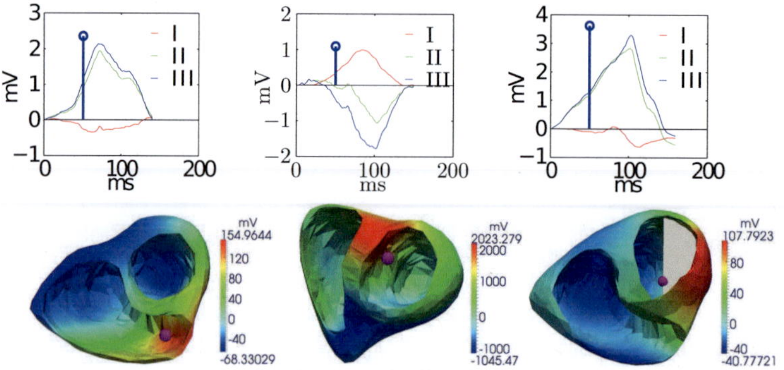

Results are not for clinical use.

Figure 7.1: ECG imaging of transmembrane voltages (TMV) in the initial phase of PVCs (blue bar) in different patients. Left-to-right: Patient 17, $\text{COMdist}_{\text{LATmin}}$=16 mm (solver: Tikhonov-2nd-order [11, 29], $\lambda = 10^{-3}$), Patient 19, $\text{COMdist}_{\text{LATmin}}$=12 mm ($\lambda = 10^{-5}$), Patient 20, $\text{COMdist}_{\text{LATmin}}$=24 mm ($\lambda = 10^{-2}$). $\text{COMdist}_{\text{LATmin}}$ is the distance of the center-of-mass of the 20% of points with greatest TMV to the earliest measured LAT. Magenta bullets mark the measured PVC origin. The time points of evaluation are marked in the upper images.

[1] There are cases where the PVC was above the MRI depicted part of the heart, so the magenta bullet may be in the blood volume of the model, e.g. for Patient 20.

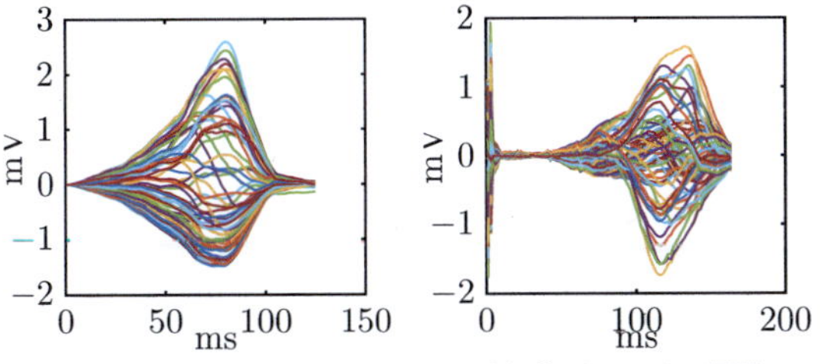

(a) PVC (b) effective pacing (EFF)

Figure 7.2: PVCs are annotated at the QRS onset. The QRS rise in effective pacings (EFF) may start long after the annotated pacing artifact.

7.1.2 Imaging of Excitation Origins

This section presents results for ECG imaging of excitation origins. I.e., ECG imaging results were either produced for an early time in the beat (for methods that produce TMVs in time) or from the ECG of the entire QRS interval (for activation time imaging methods). For the former methods, the importance of choosing a proper time of evaluation is evident, especially since PVCs and beats of effective pacings were annotated differently: one at the QRS onset, the other at the pacing artifact - which was typically long before the actual rise in the QRS, see Fig. 7.2.

Time of Evaluation

To reduce the number of variations in the study, and before comparing results of different methods, different schemes of choosing the time of evaluation were tested on two methods: Tikhonov 2nd-order (L-curve, Sect. 4.3.1, for both the BEM and FEM models) and the MAP-method (L-curve, Sect. 4.3.3, for the BEM models). The ECG is evaluated

- at 20% / 25% / 30% of the QRS length after the QRS onset (O20), (O25), (O30). QRS onset and length are annotated in the data. Percentage of QRS length is preferred over a time in ms, not to compensate for heart rate related effects (QRS duration is only slightly influenced by the RR interval [171]), but to account for the different QRS durations that ectopic beats from different origins usually have.

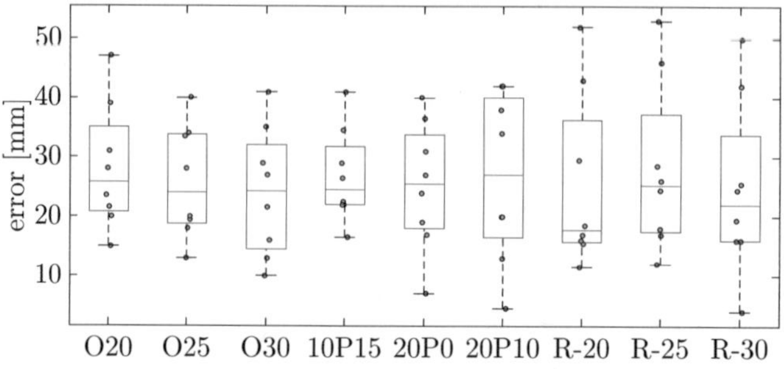

Figure 7.3: Time of evaluation (MAP, PVCs): localization error (PVCs) for imaged excitation origins (mean 95-percentile [mV] position). MAP-method (L-curve), BEM-model. Bullets represent median errors for all beats in one of the 10 patients, excluding Patient 06 and Patient 08.

- at 15% / 0% / 10% of the QRS length after the 10% / 20% / 20% R-peak amplitude (10P15), (20P0), (20P10). Absolute values of all BSPM channels are used for these definitions.
- at 20% / 25% / 30% of the QRS length before the R-peak (R-20), (R-25), (R-30). R-peaks are at the computed maximum value of the BSPM channels (absolute values).

For the MAP-method, the features were similarly computed for the simulated TMV distributions and the covariance matrices extracted from these simulations accordingly.
First, the MAP method was tested (on the BEM model). Results showed an evident preference for the R-20 scheme, see Fig. 7.3 for PVCs (clear preference) and Fig. 7.4 for effective pacings (less significant preference: among the four schemes with best medians). For a demonstration of the effects, see Fig. 7.5. Second, the same was repeated with the Tikhonov method on the BEM models and on the FEM models, see Fig. B.12 and Fig. B.13 in the Appendix for BEM (Fig. B.10 and Fig. B.11 for FEM). Results for PVCs in FEM models are indifferent and at around 30 mm median error; for effective pacings in FEM models a clear preference can be found for scheme 10P15 (median error: around 30 mm only for this scheme), and a slight preference for 20P10 and R-20; for PVCs in BEM models, results are again indifferent and at great median error level

(50 mm); for effective pacings 20P0 is the best scheme, yet at a median error of as much as 40 mm. As results show no consistent preference for any of the schemes and since the MAP method delivered much better results (median error of down to below 20 mm), the R-20 scheme was chosen for the subsequent comparison of different ECG imaging methods.

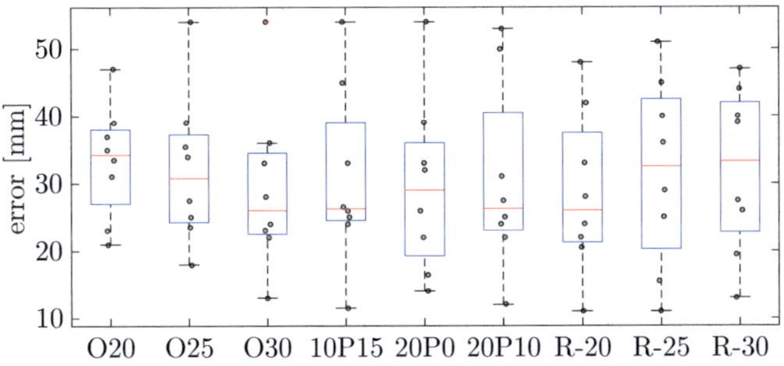

Figure 7.4: Time of evaluation (MAP, effective pacings): Localization error (effective pacings) for imaged excitation origins (mean 95-percentile [mV] position). MAP-method (L-curve), BEM-model. Bullets represent median errors for all beats in one of the 10 patients, excluding Patient 06 and Patient 08.

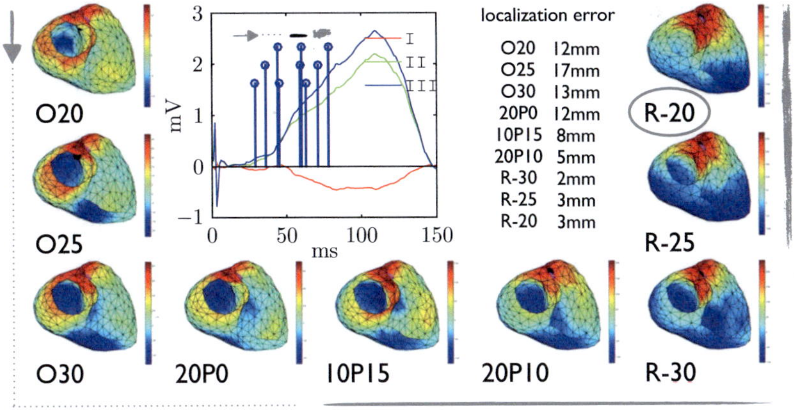

Figure 7.5: Time of evaluation schemes applied on effective beat EFFx50 of Patient 17, MAP-method (L-curve), BEM-model. Scheme R-20 was chosen for comparison of different ECG imaging methods.

Results for BEM models

Results for the BEM-models are shown in Fig. 7.6 (PVCs) and Fig. 7.7 (effective pacings). Methods for imaging TMVs as well as activation time imaging methods are tested, with the TMV imaging methods evaluated at the time of the R-20 marker:

- Methods for TMV imaging: MAP method (MAP, see Sect. 4.3.3), MAP spatio-temporal for moving window of 21ms width (MAPSTwin), MAP spatio-temporal with the SVD computed for the entire QRS (MAPSTqrs), TMV imaging with Tikhonov 2nd-order (Tikh, Sect. 4.3.1), TMV imaging using Greensite's spatio-temporal approach with the SVD computed for the entire QRS (TikhGS, Sect. 4.3.2)
- Methods for activation time imaging: critical times method with the SVD truncated at the 35th entry (CritTeff35, Sect. 4.3.5), activation time imaging using the integral method and Tikhonov 2nd-order regularization (ATintT2)

Although the critical times method (CritTeff35) performed slightly better for the effective pacings, it is clearly the MAP method without the temporal smoothing (MAP) that performed best altogether (best results for PVCs and only slightly worse than CritTeff for effective pacings).

The censoring of beats as suggested in Fig. 6.10 and Fig. 6.9 led to the following beats being excluded from evaluation:

- PVC beats: 2/4 in Patient 13
- effective pacings: 2/6 in Patient 09, 1/55 in Patient 11, 1/24 in Patient 13, 2/15 in Patient 14, 4/12 in Patient 17

I.e., the censoring only influenced the performance of a single patient for PVCs. For this patient it actually lead to an improvement by ≤ 2 mm for the MAP method, but worsened results for the CritTeff35 by ≈ 5 mm; the effect on the other methods was < 1 mm. Statistics on the effect of censoring for PVC beats are not displayed as they are considered insignificant. The effect of the censoring on the effective pacings is shown in Fig. 7.8. Although the median is zero for all methods, the percentiles - along with the outliers - clearly indicate that the censoring lead to a general increase of the localization error, except for the Tikh method, where the improvement diminishes when put into perspective of its overall error, see Fig. 7.7. The proposed censoring scheme is dropped in the following for its rather negative influence on the results. Results for the individual patients are presented in the following (Fig. 7.9 - Fig. 7.17) for the MAP method without temporal smoothing (MAP). As reference for the interpretation of localization errors, the minimum distance of the annotated excitation origin to the BEM heart mesh is displayed in the results of the PVCs in line with the values in Tab. 7.1.

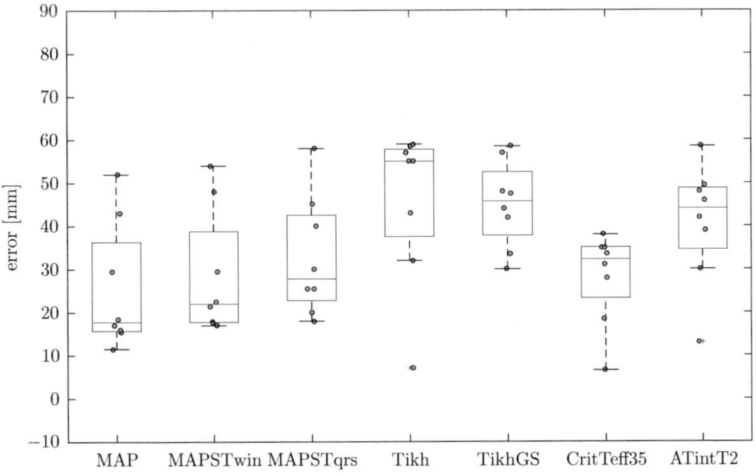

Figure 7.6: Comparison of methods (BEM-models,PVCs): results for all methods. Localization error for imaged excitation origins (mean 95-percentile [mV] position). Bullets represent median errors for all beats in one of the 10 patients, excluding Patient 06 and Patient 08.

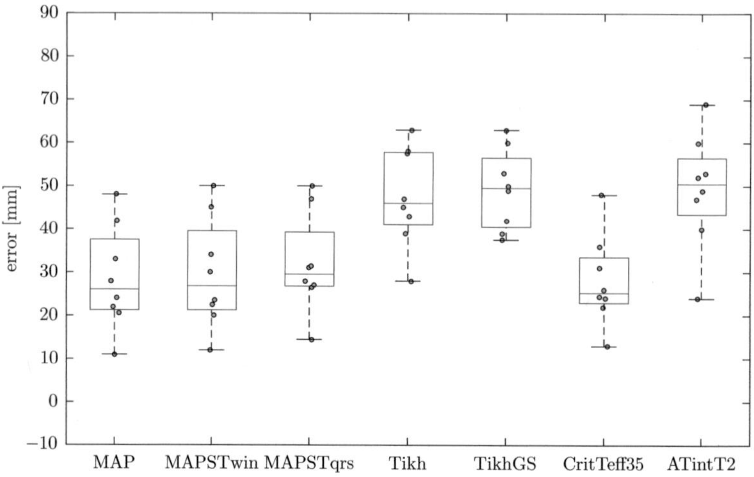

Figure 7.7: Comparison of methods (BEM-models, effective pacings): results for all methods. Localization error for imaged excitation origins (mean 95-percentile [mV] position). Bullets represent median errors for all beats in one of the 10 patients, excluding Patient 06 and Patient 08.

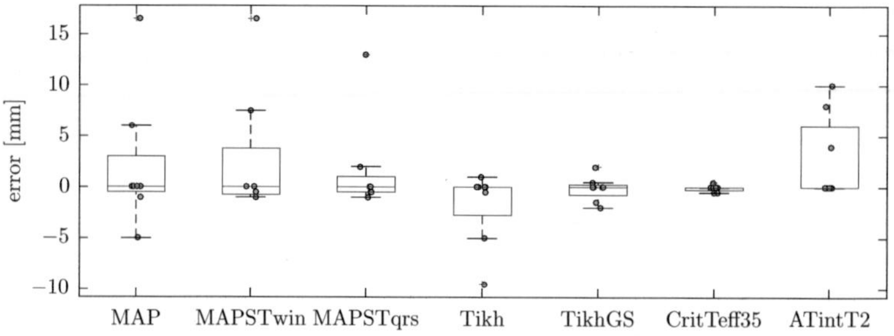

Figure 7.8: Effect of the censoring on localization errors (BEM-models, effective pacings), results for all methods. Bullets represent the difference between median errors for all beats in one of the 10 patients, excluding Patient 06 and Patient 08. The difference is computed with respect to the unscensored results in Fig. 7.7.

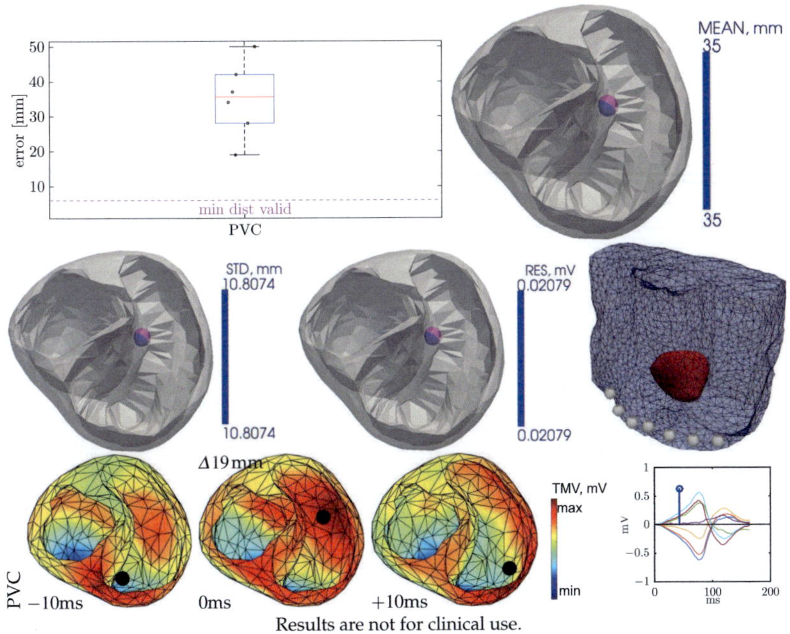

Figure 7.9: Results for Patient 06 (BEM-model, MAP method, localization error for imaged excitation origins (mean 95-percentile [mV] position). All PVC beats (n=6) that had been annotated in the study are represented as bullets. The imaged excitation spread is shown for 3 time steps of the best beat in the boxplot of the PVC (black: imaged origin, magenta: measured origin). Localization error: MEAN, STD; mean of $\|Ax - b\|_2$: RES; min dist valid: distance of the measured excitation origin to the closest point in the heart mesh. Effective pacings are not available for this patient. (Presentation of data is enabled with Paraview [172].) (Since there is only one single validation measurement, the heart plots only display the MEAN, STD and mean residual of beats from a single point.)

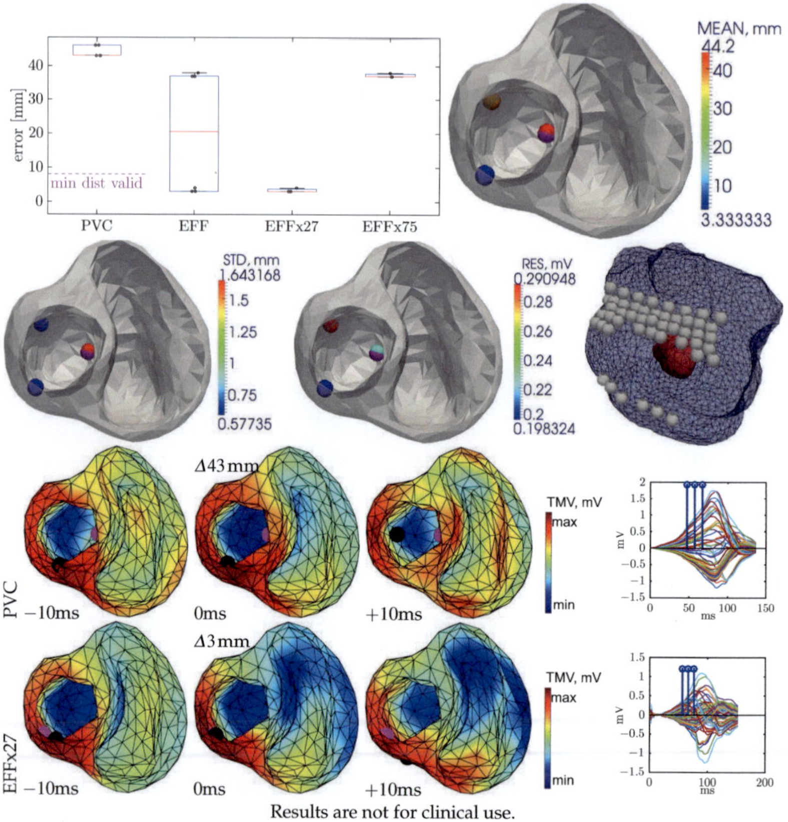

Figure 7.10: Results for Patient 09 (BEM-model, MAP method, localization error for imaged excitation origins (mean 95-percentile [mV] position). All PVC beats (n=5) and effective pacings (n=6, EFF) that had been annotated in the study are represented as bullets. Beats from pacing positions 27 (n=3) and 75 (n=3) are also displayed separately as EFFx27 and EFFx75. The imaged excitation spread is shown for 3 time steps of the best beat in the boxplots of the PVC and of EFFx27 (black: imaged origin, magenta: measured origin). Localization error: MEAN, STD; mean of $\|Ax-b\|_2$: RES; min dist valid: distance of the measured excitation origin to the closest point in the heart mesh.

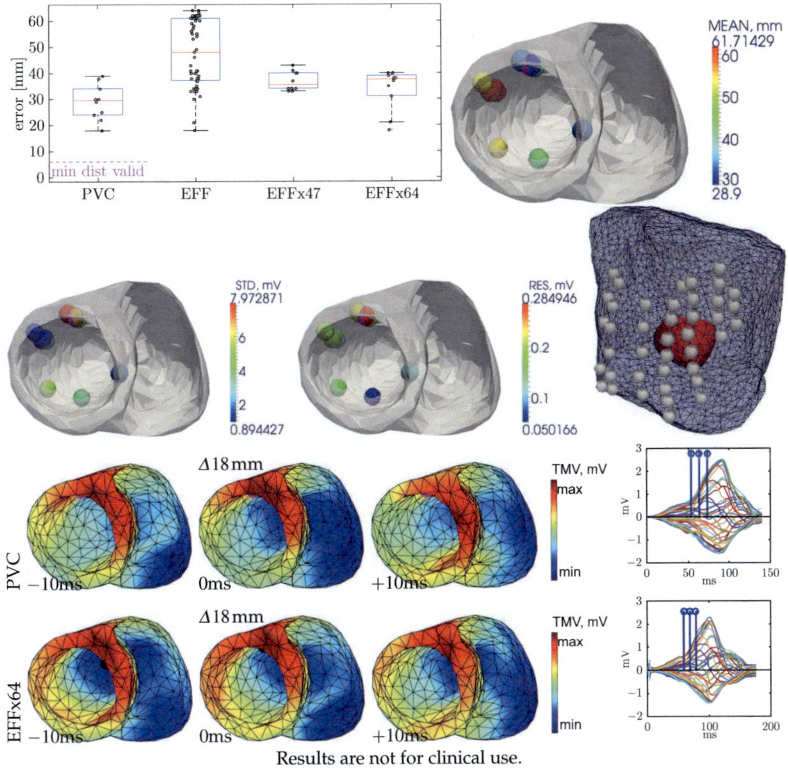

Figure 7.11: Results for Patient 11 (BEM-model, MAP method, localization error for imaged excitation origins (mean 95-percentile [mV] position). All PVC beats (n=10) and effective pacings (n=55, EFF) that had been annotated in the study are represented as bullets. Beats from pacing positions 47 (n=10) and 64 (n=10) are also displayed separately as EFFx47 and EFFx64. The imaged excitation spread is shown for 3 time steps of the best beat in the boxplots of the PVC and of EFFx64 (black: imaged origin, magenta: measured origin). Localization error: MEAN, STD; mean of $\|Ax-b\|_2$: RES; min dist valid: distance of the measured excitation origin to the closest point in the heart mesh.

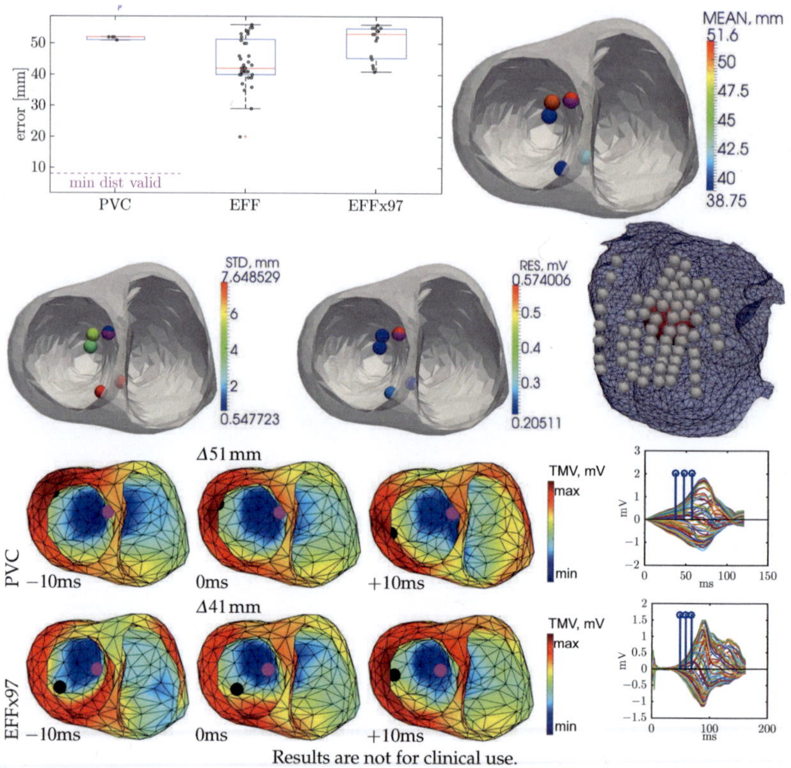

Figure 7.12: Results for Patient 12 (BEM-model, MAP method, localization error for imaged excitation origins (mean 95-percentile [mV] position). All PVC beats (n=5) and effective pacings (n=37, EFF) that had been annotated in the study are represented as bullets. Beats from pacing position 97 (n=15) are also displayed separately as EFFx97. The imaged excitation spread is shown for 3 time steps of the best beat in the boxplots of the PVC and of EFFx97 (black: imaged origin, magenta: measured origin). Localization error: MEAN, STD; mean of $\|Ax-b\|_2$: RES; min dist valid: distance of the measured excitation origin to the closest point in the heart mesh.

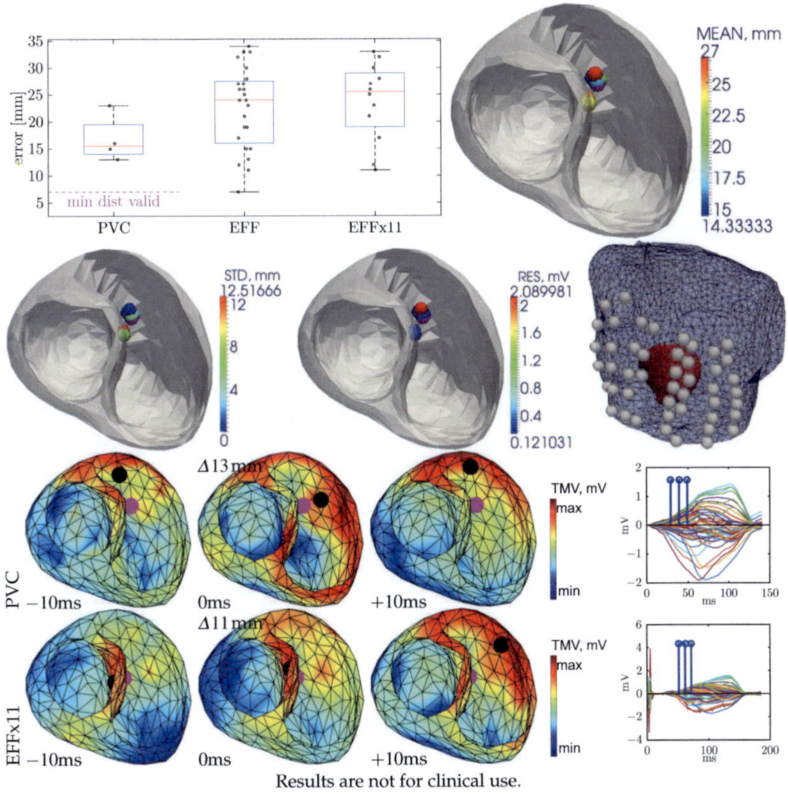

Figure 7.13: Results for Patient 13 (BEM-model, MAP method, localization error for imaged excitation origins (mean 95-percentile [mV] position). All PVC beats (n=4) and effective pacings (n=24, EFF) that had been annotated in the study are represented as bullets. Beats from pacing position 11 (n=12) are also displayed separately as EFFx11. The imaged excitation spread is shown for 3 time steps of the best beat in the boxplots of the PVC and of EFFx11 (black: imaged origin, magenta: measured origin). Localization error: MEAN, STD; mean of $\|Ax-b\|_2$: RES; min dist valid: distance of the measured excitation origin to the closest point in the heart mesh.

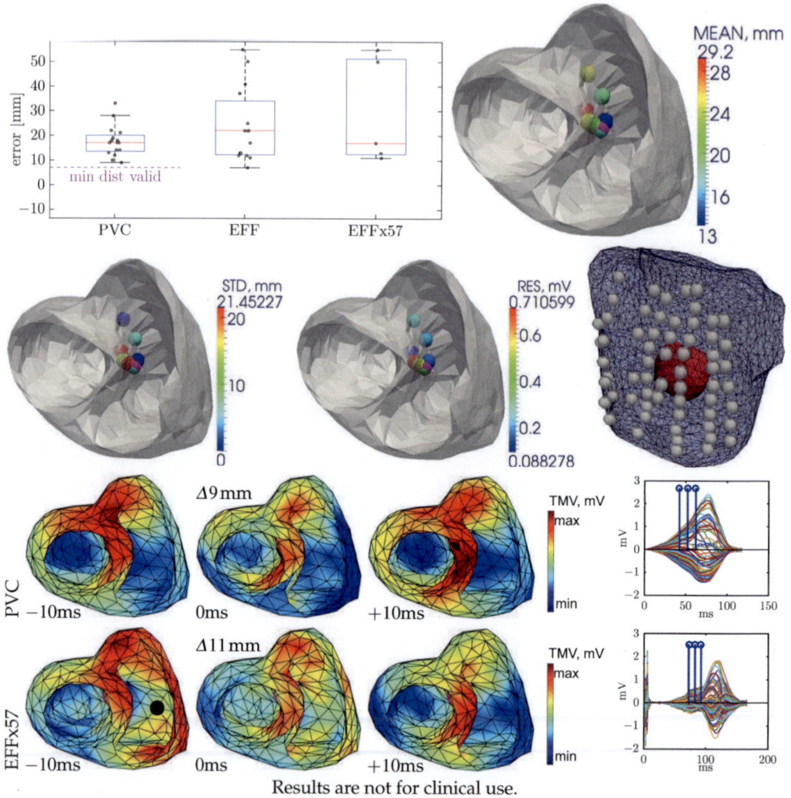

Figure 7.14: Results for Patient 14 (BEM-model, MAP method, localization error for imaged excitation origins (mean 95-percentile [mV] position). All PVC beats (n=16) and effective pacings (n=15, EFF) that had been annotated in the study are represented as bullets. Beats from pacing position 57 (n=5) are also displayed separately as EFFx57. The imaged excitation spread is shown for 3 time steps of the best beat in the boxplots of the PVC and of EFFx57 (black: imaged origin, magenta: measured origin). Localization error: MEAN, STD; mean of $\|Ax-b\|_2$: RES; min dist valid: distance of the measured excitation origin to the closest point in the heart mesh.

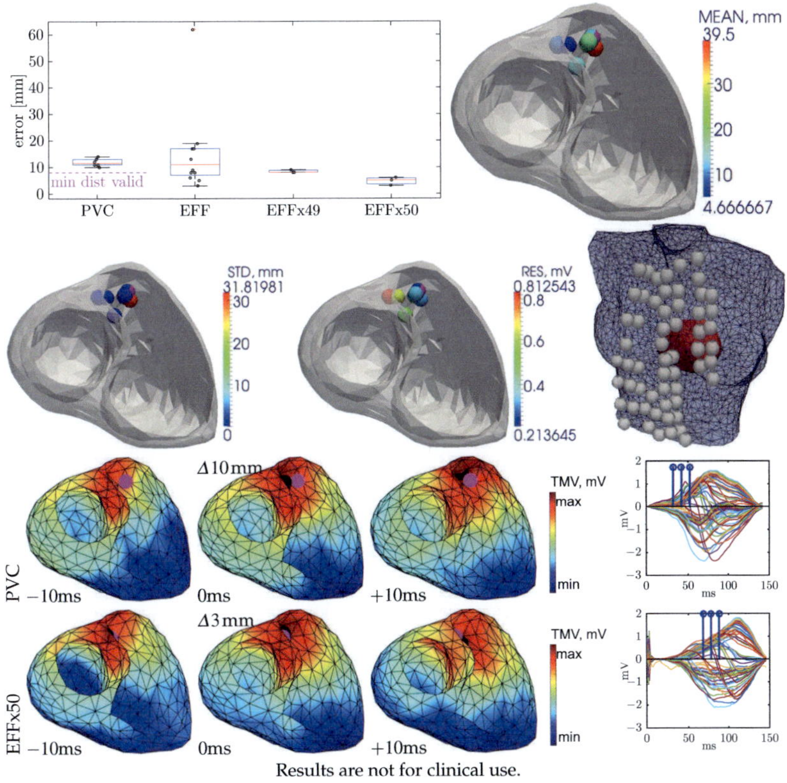

Figure 7.15: Results for Patient 17 (BEM-model, MAP method, localization error for imaged excitation origins (mean 95-percentile [mV] position). All PVC beats (n=6) and effective pacings (n=12, EFF) that had been annotated in the study are represented as bullets. Beats from pacing positions 49 (n=3) and 50 (n=3) are also displayed separately as EFFx49 and EFFx50. The imaged excitation spread is shown for 3 time steps of the best beat in the boxplots of the PVC and of EFFx50 (black: imaged origin, magenta: measured origin). Localization error: MEAN, STD; mean of $\|Ax-b\|_2$: RES; min dist valid: distance of the measured excitation origin to the closest point in the heart mesh.

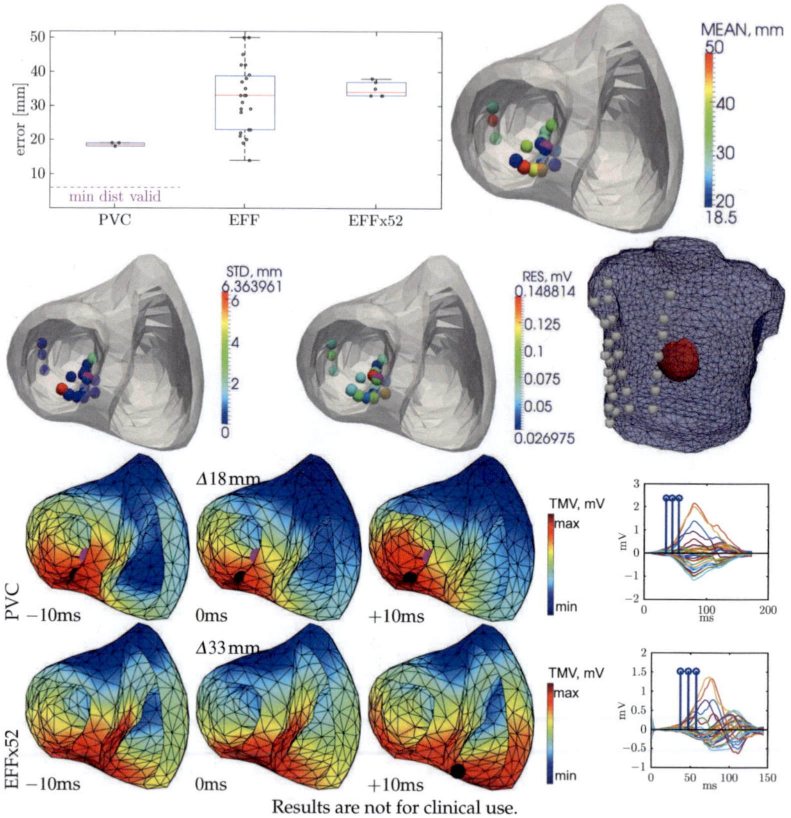

Figure 7.16: Results for Patient 19 (BEM-model, MAP method, localization error for imaged excitation origins (mean 95-percentile [mV] position). All PVC beats (n=4) and effective pacings (n=23, EFF) that had been annotated in the study are represented as bullets. Beats from pacing position 52 (n=6) are also displayed separately as EFFx52. The imaged excitation spread is shown for 3 time steps of the best beat in the boxplots of the PVC and of EFFx52 (black: imaged origin, magenta: measured origin). Localization error: MEAN, STD; mean of $||Ax - b||_2$: RES; min dist valid: distance of the measured excitation origin to the closest point in the heart mesh.

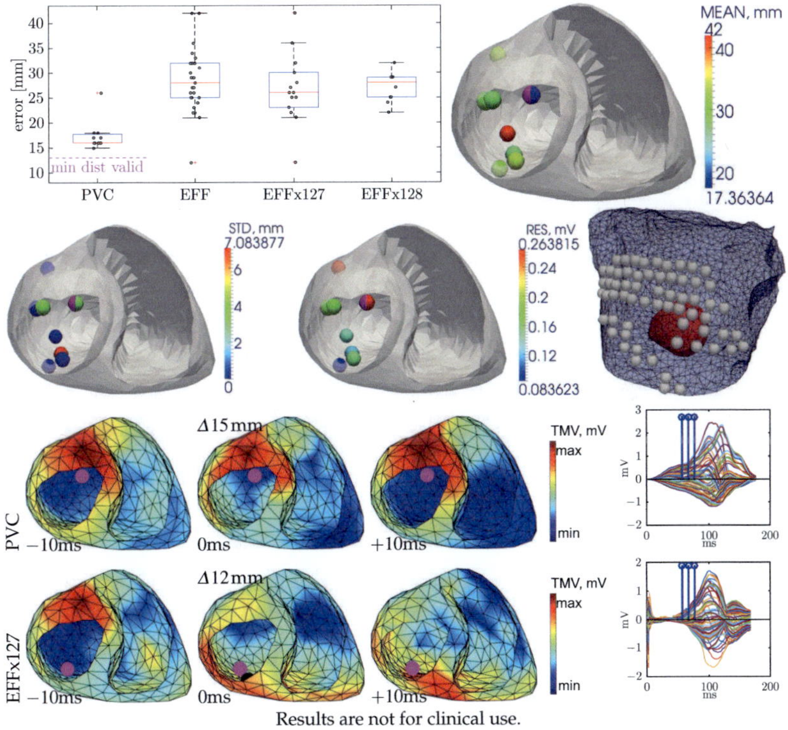

Figure 7.17: Results for Patient 20 (BEM-model, MAP method, localization error for imaged excitation origins (mean 95-percentile [mV] position). All PVC beats (n=11) and effective pacings (n=29, EFF) that had been annotated in the study are represented as bullets. Beats from pacing positions 127 (n=14) and 128 (n=10) are also displayed separately as EFFx127 and EFFx128. The imaged excitation spread is shown for 3 time steps of the best beat in the boxplots of the PVC and of EFFx127 (black: imaged origin, magenta: measured origin). Localization error: MEAN, STD; mean of $\|Ax-b\|_2$: RES; min dist valid: distance of the measured excitation origin to the closest point in the heart mesh.

Results for FEM models

For the FEM models, methods for imaging TMVs as well as activation time imaging methods are tested again, but now also against a model-based approach:

- Methods for TMV imaging (evaluated at R-20, according to the results for BEM): MAP method (MAP, Sect. 4.3.3), MAP spatio-temporal for moving window of 21ms width (MAPSTwin), MAP spatio-temporal with the SVD computed for the entire QRS (MAPSTqrs), TMV imaging with Tikhonov 2nd-order, L-curve method (Tikh LC, Sect. 4.3.1)
- Methods for activation time imaging: activation time imaging with the integral method (ATintT2, Sect. 4.3.4, L-curve)
- Model-based approaches: computation of similarities between model-based ECG simulations and the measured ECG, see Sect. 5.5, with either the mean temporal (MODcct) or mean spatial correlation coefficient serving as similarity measure (MODccs).

For Tikhonov regularization (2nd order, L-curve), it is known that the L-curve method does not always identify the ideal regularization parameter; yet, the CRESO method, which is an alternative, did not deliver notably different results when applied on sample datasets. There is, however, a common practical suggestion that for repeated studies with the same setup the ideal regularization parameter can be known from experience. To test for this hypothesis, the study with the TMV imaging method was repeated for a range of parameter values while the R-20 scheme was used to pick the time of evaluation. Fig. B.14 and Fig. B.15 in the Attachment reveal that a regularization parameter of 10^{-6} is best for the PVCs; however, for effective pacings, a regularization parameter of 10^{-3} can be considered the best choice across patients. Effective pacings are more frequent in the study. A variant with a preset regularization parameter of 10^{-3} is therefore included in the final comparison of methods on the FEM model (Tikh -3).
Results for PVCs are given in Fig. 7.18 and for effective pacings in Fig. 7.19. It is revealed that for PVCs, most good solutions are found with the MODcct method. For effective pacings, however, it is the

MODccs method. Results are thus inconsistent over different types of beats – regarding the medians of median patient-wise errors. Therefore and since the results are short of those of the BEM models at least for the PVCs, practical considerations are used to motivate the further evaluation and presentation of results. It is assumed that only at $\leq 2\,\text{cm}$ median error results are of value for clinical applications. The most such results are obtained with the MODcct method (4 cases for PVCs and 2 cases for effective pacings), whereas it is 2 and 2 for the MODccs method. In the discussion (Chapt. 8) it will be studied where these results occur and whether the good results are obtained for the same patients as previously with the BEM-based models, with the intention to reveal the effect of modeling errors as opposed to intrinsic errors of the methods. Results for the MODcct approach are presented in the following for each patient individually.

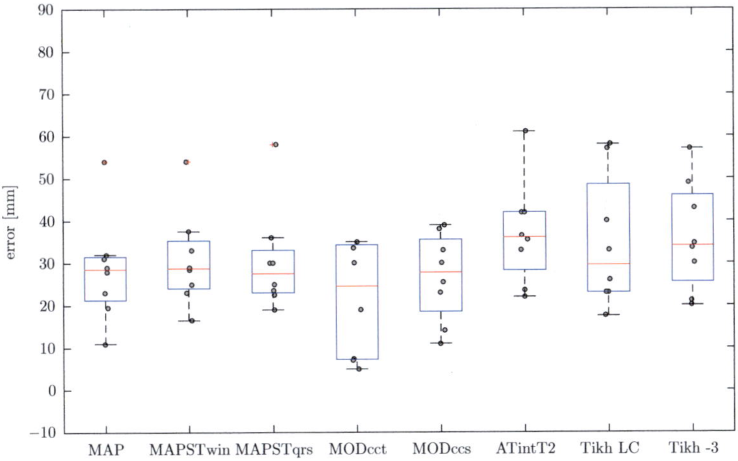

Figure 7.18: Comparison of methods (FEM-models, PVCs): results for all methods. Localization error for imaged excitation origins (mean 95-percentile [mV] position). Bullets represent median errors for all beats in one of the 10 patients, excluding Patient 06 and Patient 08. MAP: maximum a posteriori based regularization; MAPSTwin: spatio-temporal variant with window; MAPSTqrs: spatio-temporal variant applied on entire QRS; ATintT2: activation time imaging with the integral method (Tikhonov 2nd-order); TikhR-3: Tikhonov 2nd-order regularization, $\lambda = 10^{-3}$; TikhLV: Tikhonov regularization, L-curve.

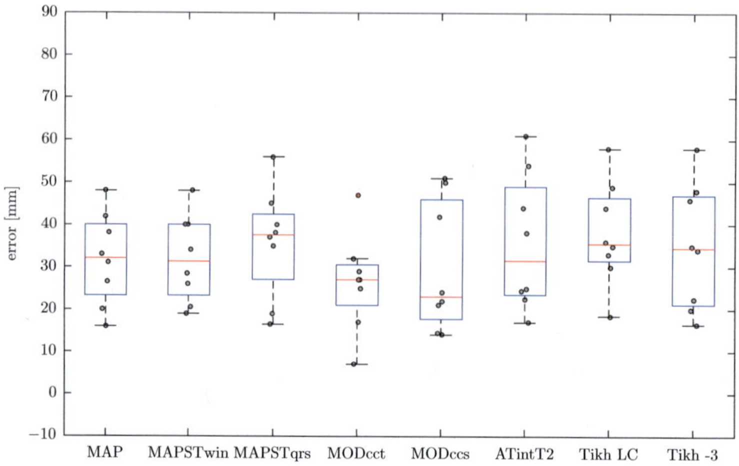

Figure 7.19: Comparison of methods (FEM-models, effective pacings): results for all methods. Localization error for imaged excitation origins (mean 95-percentile [mV] position). Bullets represent median errors for all beats in one of the 10 patients, excluding Patient 06 and Patient 08. MAP: maximum a posteriori based regularization; MAPSTwin: spatio-temporal variant with window; MAPSTqrs: spatio-temporal variant applied on entire QRS; ATintT2: activation time imaging with the integral method (Tikhonov 2nd-order); TikhR-3: Tikhonov 2nd-order regularization, $\lambda = 10^{-3}$; TikhLV: Tikhonov regularization, L-curve.

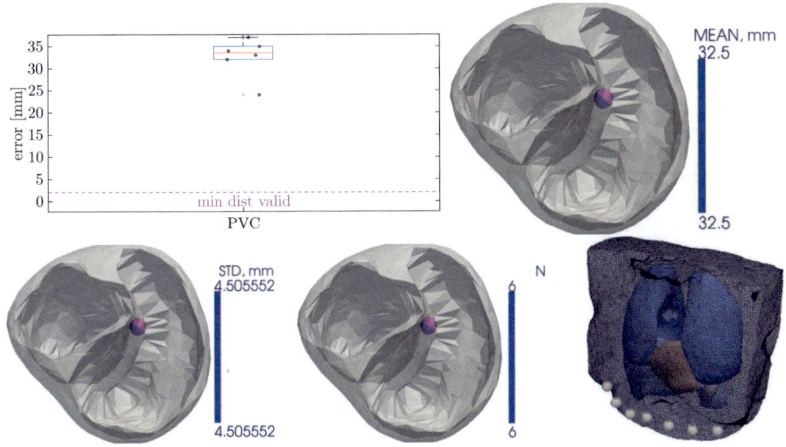

Figure 7.20: Results for Patient 06 (FEM-model, MODcct method, localization error for imaged excitation origins (mean 95-percentile [mV] position). All PVC beats (n=6) that had been annotated in the study are represented as bullets; effective pacings are not available for this patient. Localization error: MEAN, STD; N: number of measurements; min dist valid: distance of the measured excitation origin to the closest point in the heart mesh. (Since there is only one single validation measurement, the heart plots only display the MEAN, STD and mean residual of beats from a single point.)

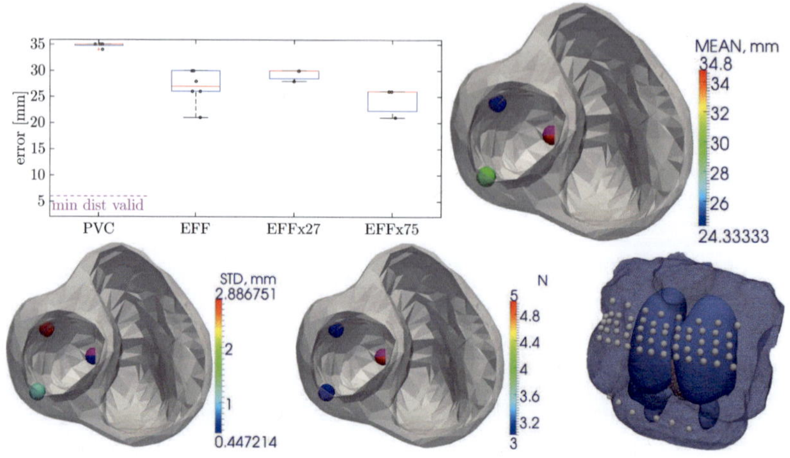

Figure 7.21: Results for Patient 09 (FEM-model, MODcct method, localization error for imaged excitation origins (mean 95-percentile [mV] position). All PVC beats (n=5) and effective pacings (n=6, EFF) that had been annotated in the study are represented as bullets. Beats from pacing positions 27 (n=3) and 75 (n=3) are also displayed separately as EFFx27 and EFFx75. Localization error: MEAN, STD; N: number of measurements; min dist valid: distance of the measured excitation origin to the closest point in the heart mesh.

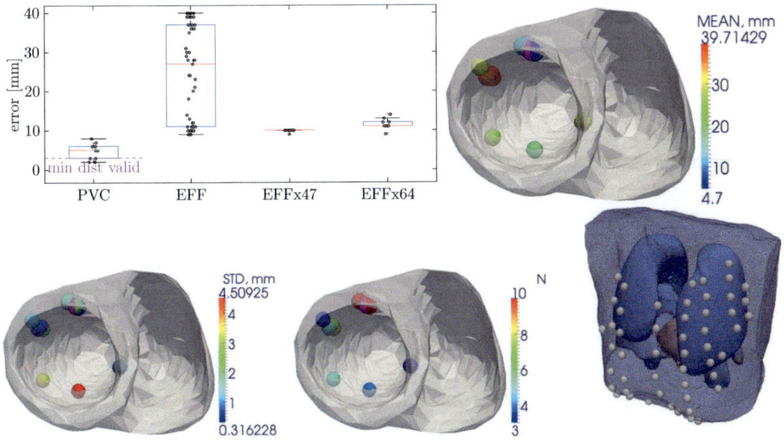

Figure 7.22: Results for Patient 11 (FEM-model, MODcct method, localization error for imaged excitation origins (mean 95-percentile [mV] position). All PVC beats (n=10) and effective pacings (n=55, EFF) that had been annotated in the study are represented as bullets. Beats from pacing positions 47 (n=10) and 64 (n=10) are also displayed separately as EFFx47 and EFFx64. Localization error: MEAN, STD; N: number of measurements; min dist valid: distance of the measured excitation origin to the closest point in the heart mesh.

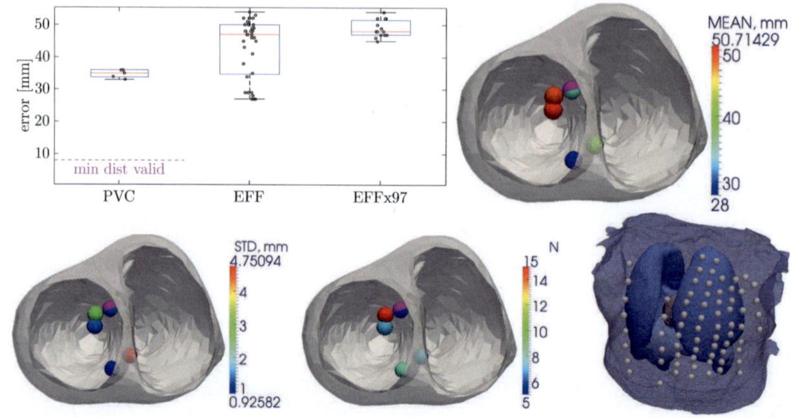

Figure 7.23: Results for Patient 12 (FEM-model, MODcct method, localization error for imaged excitation origins (mean 95-percentile [mV] position). All PVC beats (n=5) and effective pacings (n=37, EFF) that had been annotated in the study are represented as bullets. Beats from pacing position 97 (n=15) are also displayed separately as EFFx97. Localization error: MEAN, STD; N: number of measurements; min dist valid: distance of the measured excitation origin to the closest point in the heart mesh.

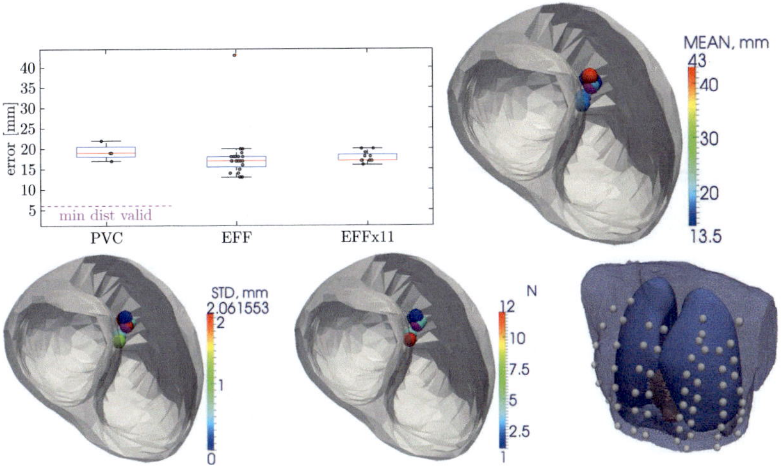

Figure 7.24: Results for Patient 13 (FEM-model, MODcct method, localization error for imaged excitation origins (mean 95-percentile [mV] position). All PVC beats (n=4) and effective pacings (n=24, EFF) that had been annotated in the study are represented as bullets. Beats from pacing position 11 (n=12) are also displayed separately as EFFx11. Localization error: MEAN, STD; N: number of measurements; min dist valid: distance of the measured excitation origin to the closest point in the heart mesh.

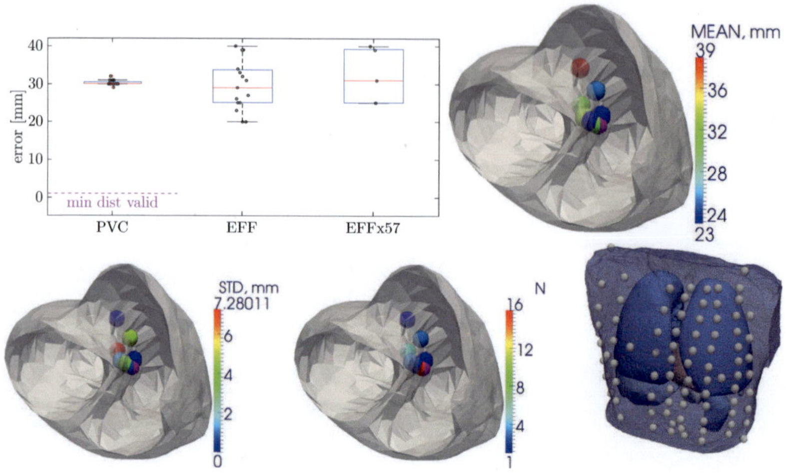

Figure 7.25: Results for Patient 14 (FEM-model, MODcct method, localization error for imaged excitation origins (mean 95-percentile [mV] position). All PVC beats (n=16) and effective pacings (n=15, EFF) that had been annotated in the study are represented as bullets. Beats from pacing position 57 (n=5) are also displayed separately as EFFx57. Localization error: MEAN, STD; N: number of measurements; min dist valid: distance of the measured excitation origin to the closest point in the heart mesh.

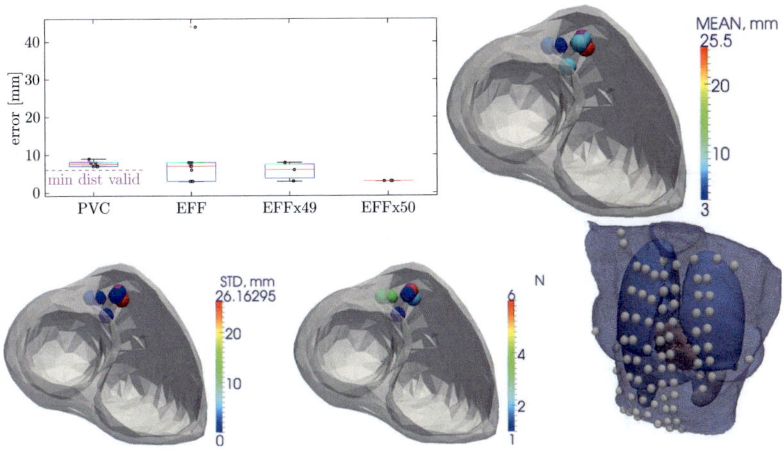

Figure 7.26: Results for Patient 17 (FEM-model, MODcct method, localization error for imaged excitation origins (mean 95-percentile [mV] position). All PVC beats (n=6) and effective pacings (n=12, EFF) that had been annotated in the study are represented as bullets. Beats from pacing positions 49 (n=3) and 50 (n=3) are also displayed separately as EFFx49 and EFFx50. Localization error: MEAN, STD; N: number of measurements; min dist valid: distance of the measured excitation origin to the closest point in the heart mesh.

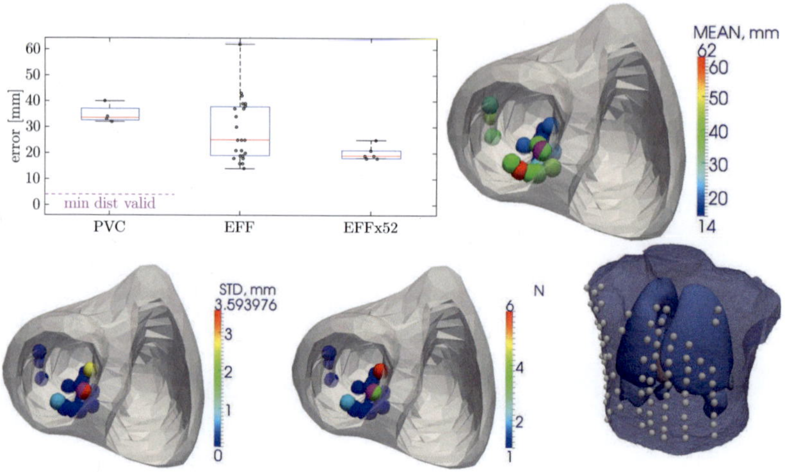

Figure 7.27: Results for Patient 19 (FEM-model, MODcct method, localization error for imaged excitation origins (mean 95-percentile [mV] position). All PVC beats (n=4) and effective pacings (n=23, EFF) that had been annotated in the study are represented as bullets. Beats from pacing position 52 (n=6) are also displayed separately as EFFx52. Localization error: MEAN, STD; N: number of measurements; min dist valid: distance of the measured excitation origin to the closest point in the heart mesh.

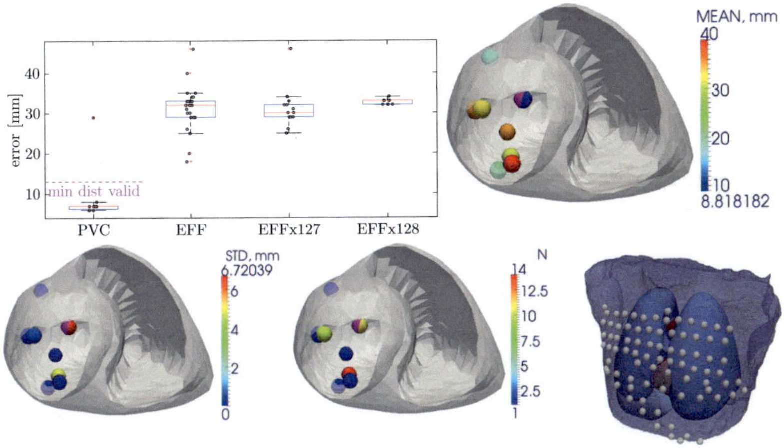

Figure 7.28: Results for Patient 20 (FEM-model, MODcct method, localization error for imaged excitation origins (mean 95-percentile [mV] position). All PVC beats (n=11) and effective pacings (n=29, EFF) that had been annotated in the study are represented as bullets. Beats from pacing positions 127 (n=14) and 128 (n=10) are also displayed separately as EFFx127 and EFFx128. Localization error: MEAN, STD; N: number of measurements; min dist valid: distance of the measured excitation origin to the closest point in the heart mesh.

Effect of Averaging Multiple Beats

For the MAP-method (and the R-20 scheme) it was tested whether the averaging of multiple beats has an effect on the quality of results, see Fig. 7.29. Beats of the same origin were averaged and then introduced in the statistics as multiple identical copies; hence, the original number of beats and the composition of the statistics did not change. The effect of the averaging (averaged PVC beats: PVCAV, averaged effective pacings: EFFAV) was in the range of a millimeter on the median error of the patient-wise results. There were, however, effects on the individual patient results where the median localization error was reduced by a few millimeters for both PVCs and effective pacings (e.g. for Patient 14, which is shown in Fig. 7.29). Fig. 7.29(c) depicts how the averaging of the 16 PVC beats in Patient 14 results in a smoothed averaged beat PVCAV. The representation of these averaged beats is clearly reflected in the statistics of Patient 14, see Fig. 7.29(b).

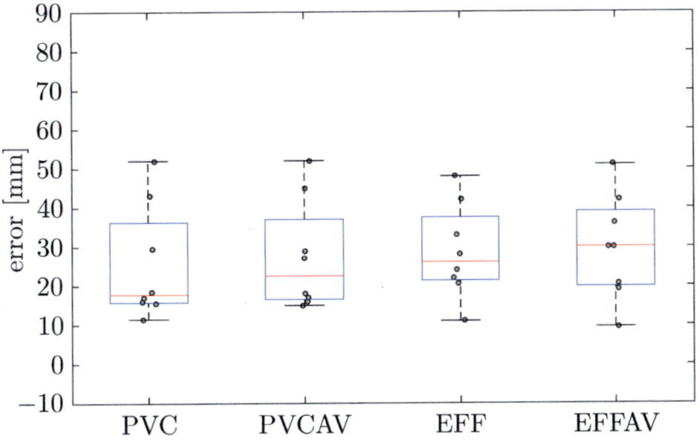

(a) all patients

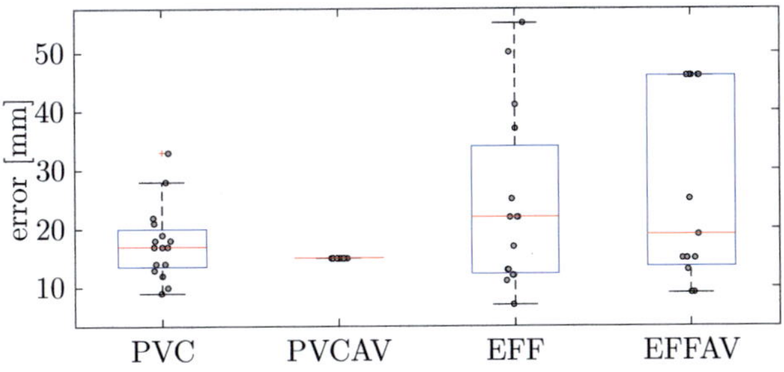

(b) Patient 14

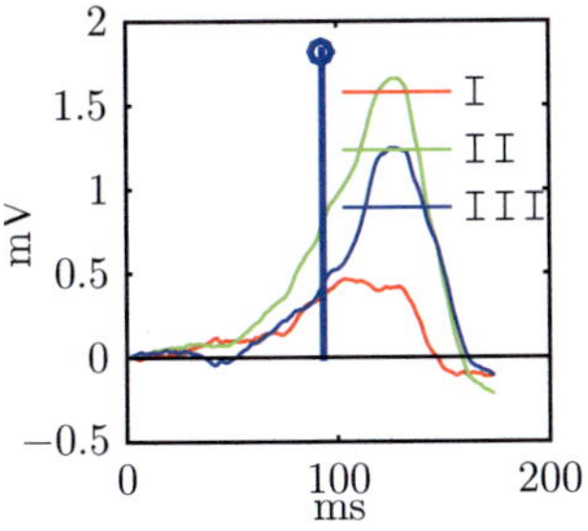

(c) Patient 14 (single PVC beat)

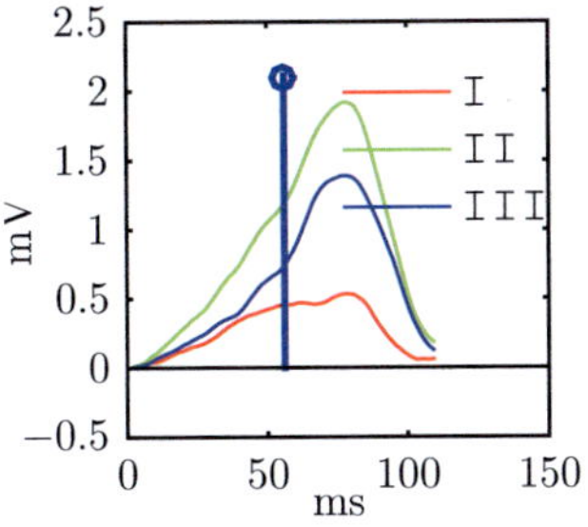

(d) Patient 14 (averaged: PVCAV)

Figure 7.29: Results for averaged beats (MAP, BEM-model): Localization error for imaged excitation origins (mean 95-percentile [mV] position). Bullets in (a) represent median errors for all beats in one of the 10 patients, excluding Patient 06 and Patient 08. Bullet in (b) represent single beats. EFF: effective pacings; EFFAV: EFF, averaged; PVCAV: PVC, averaged.

7.1.3 Imaging of Activation Times

For the validation of imaged activation times, a case study is shown as introduction to the section, see Fig. 7.30. Activation time imaging is demonstrated here with the disciplined convex programming framework from Sect. 5.3 that, in addition to a solution with the Tikhonov integral method ATintT2 (Fig. 7.30(a)), which is called LCλ5 in this context, introduces a-priori knowledge from a random set of 22 of the 65 available LAT samples (b) and then all 65 available measurements in the LAT map (c). In the example, the regularization parameter is tuned with the L-curve method and an upper boundary for the root mean square error with respect to the provided activation times of $\eta = 5\,\text{ms}$ is chosen. The root mean squared error (RMSE) of the activation times was 33.0 ms for the ATintT2 method and decreased to 13.6 ms and 5 ms when 22 or all of 65 available LAT measurements were introduced in the solution. The distance to the earliest measured LAT was 24 ms without a-priori knowledge, reduced to 16 ms with knowledge of 22 out of 65 measurements and increased again to 23 ms with knowledge of all 65 measurements.
This reveals substantial information on the quality measure used in the localization of excitation origins. Fig 7.31 shows the 5th percentile of the imaged activation times (red), the average position of which is marked with a black spot. The location of the earliest measured LAT is shown in magenta. While the distance of the excitation origin to the modeled endocardium is obvious (distance to the FEM heart mesh is 13 mm), it is also revealed in Fig. 7.30 that the solution with 16 mm distance is indeed closer to the actual excitation origin when looking at the distribution of TMVs in the myocardial wall - as opposed to the solution with full knowledge of the local activation times. This rises the question whether the earliest activation time in the electroanatomical map is indeed close to the mean position of the early local activation times and whether the mean position of the earliest local activation times should not be chosen as the validation reference instead (see discussion in Sect. 8).
The same study (activation time imaging framework from Sect. 5.3) was repeated for all patients with validation measurements available.

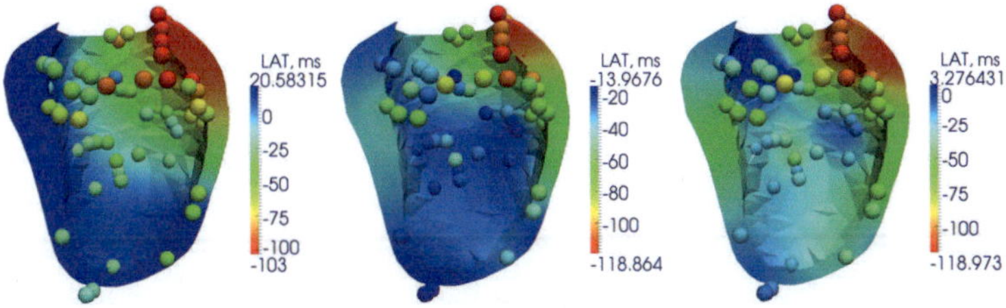

(a) ATintT2, $RMSE_{65} = 33.0$ms (b) A-priori: 22 of 65 LATs, $RMSE_{65} = 13.6$ms (c) A-priori: 65 of 65 LATs, $RMSE_{65} = 5.0$ms

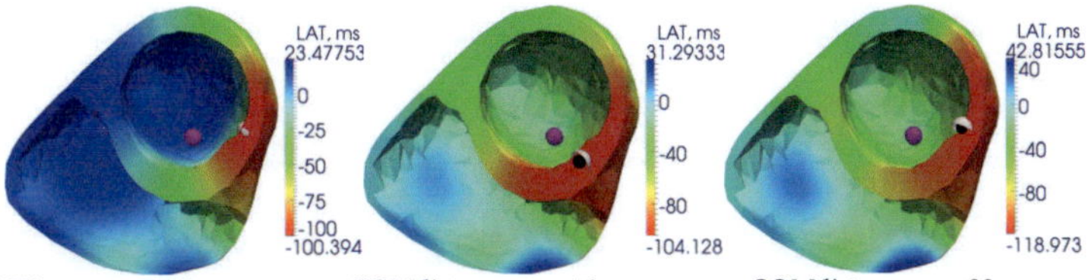

$COMdist_{\text{LATmin}} = 24\,mm$ $COMdist_{\text{LATmin}} = 16\,mm$ $COMdist_{\text{LATmin}} = 23\,mm$

Figure 7.30: Activation time imaging (Patient 20). The method in [41, 42] is used (a) and embedded in a disciplined convex programming framework (see Sect. 5.3) to introduce a random set of LAT samples (b) and then all available measurements (c). $\lambda = \lambda(\text{L-curve}), \eta = 5\,\text{ms}$. The root mean squared error (RMSE) is computed with respect to the available LAT measurements (Fig. B.9). The distance of the center-of-mass of the earliest 5% of activated points (black spot with white circumsphere) is computed with respect to the earliest measured LAT (magenta spot) as $\text{COMdist}_{\text{LATmin}}$.

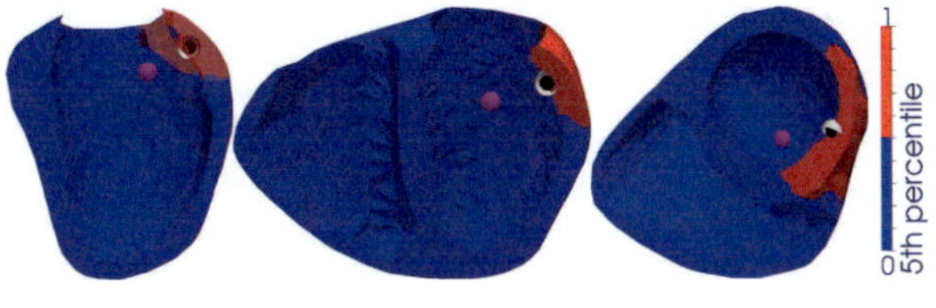

Figure 7.31: Earliest activated points in Fig. 7.30(c) (result with all available measurements): average location of 5th percentile (black spot with white circumsphere) with respect to the earliest measured LAT (magenta spot).

Patient 06 was excluded from the study for the little number of available measurements, Patient 13 was excluded as the activation time map shows measurements of normal sinus rhythm. A-priori knowledge was introduced from approximately 25% of the available measurements (P) or all available measurements (A). Measurements for the former approach were chosen pseudo-randomly at a 0.25 probability rate and stored for each patient to not influence the comparison of methods.

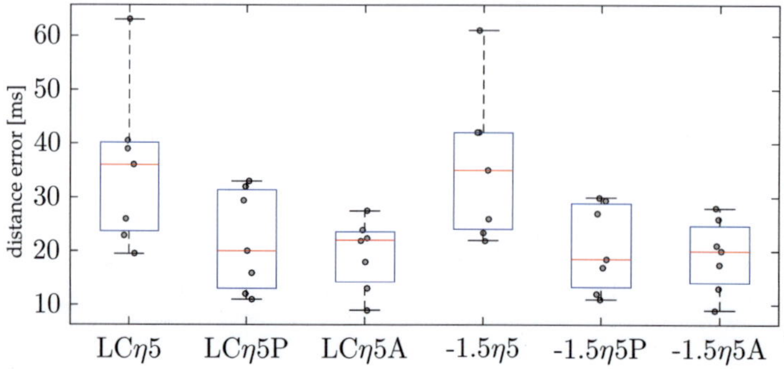

Figure 7.32: Imaging of Activation Times with and without knowledge from measurements (FEM-models, PVCs): results for all methods. Localization error for imaged excitation origins (mean 5-percentile [ms] position). Bullets represent median errors for all beats in one of the 10 patients, excluding Patient 06, Patient 08 and Patient 13. LC: λ is chosen using the L-curve method, -1.5: $\lambda = 10^{-1.5}$, η5: $\eta = 5$, P: a-priori knowledge from $\approx 25\%$ of the available measurements, A: all available measurements used as a-priori knowledge.

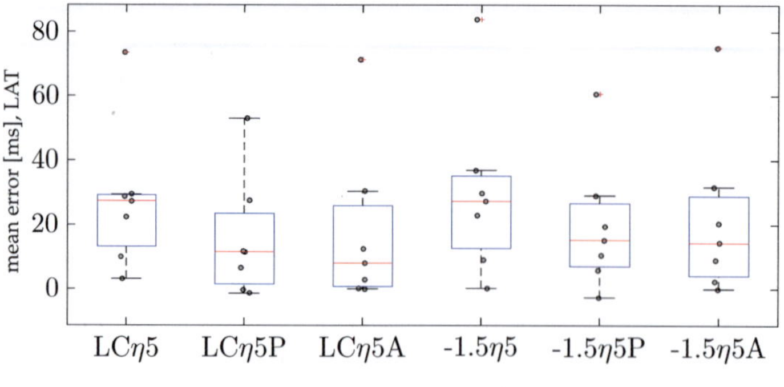

Figure 7.33: Imaging of Activation Times with and without knowledge from measurements (FEM-models, PVCs): results for all methods. Mean error with respect to the measured LATs [ms]. Bullets represent median errors for all beats in one of the 10 patients, excluding Patient 06, Patient 08 and Patient 13. LC: λ is chosen using the L-curve method, -1.5: $\lambda = 10^{-1.5}$, η5: $\eta = 5$,P: a-priori knowledge from $\approx 25\%$ of the available measurements, A: all available measurements used as a-priori knowledge.

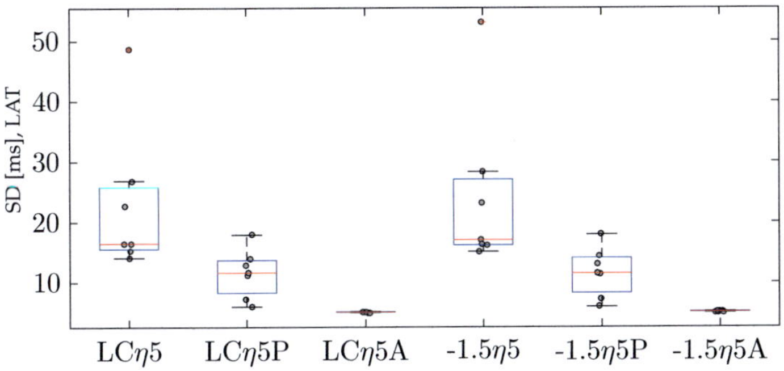

Figure 7.34: Imaging of Activation Times with and without knowledge from measurements (FEM-models, PVCs): results for all methods. Standard deviation of the error with respect to the measured LATs [ms]. Bullets represent median errors for all beats in one of the 10 patients, excluding Patient 06, Patient 08 and Patient 13. LC: λ is chosen using the L-curve method, -1.5: $\lambda = 10^{-1.5}$, $\eta 5$: $\eta = 5$, P: a-priori knowledge from $\approx 25\%$ of the available measurements, A: all available measurements used as a-priori knowledge.

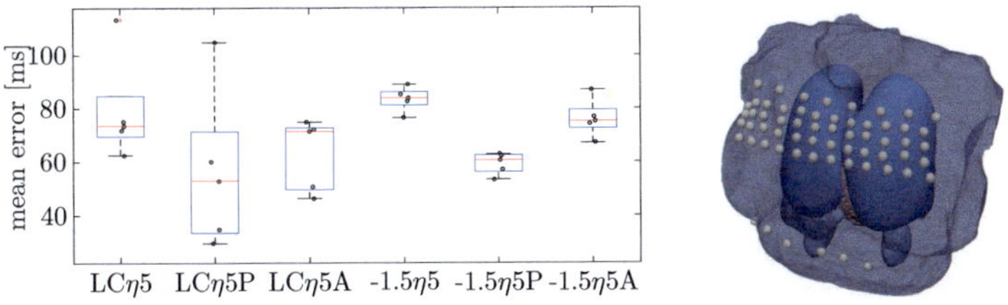

Figure 7.35: Results for Patient 09 (FEM-model), imaging of activation times with and without knowledge from measurements, error with respect to measured LATs (mean [ms]). Bullets represent single PVC beats (n=5). P: a-priori knowledge from 14 ($\approx 25\%$) of the 31 available measurements (built from 39 CARTO LATs), A: all available measurements used as a-priori knowledge.

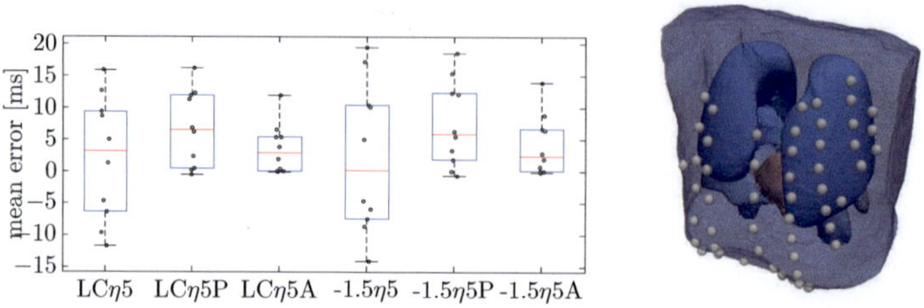

Figure 7.36: Results for Patient 11 (FEM-model), imaging of activation times with and without knowledge from measurements, error with respect to measured LATs (mean [ms]). Bullets represent single PVC beats (n=10). P: a-priori knowledge from 14 ($\approx 25\%$) of the 35 available measurements (built from 65 CARTO LATs), A: all available measurements used as a-priori knowledge.

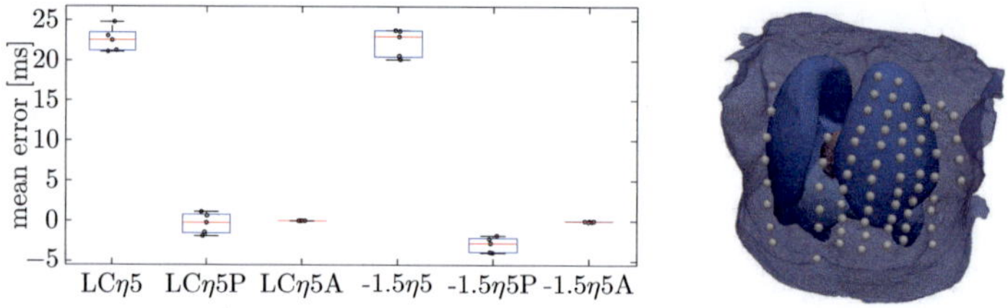

Figure 7.37: Results for Patient 12 (FEM-model), imaging of activation times with and without knowledge from measurements, error with respect to measured LATs (mean [ms]). Bullets represent single PVC beats (n=5). P: a-priori knowledge from 23 ($\approx 25\%$) of the 67 available measurements (built from 82 CARTO LATs), A: all available measurements used as a-priori knowledge.

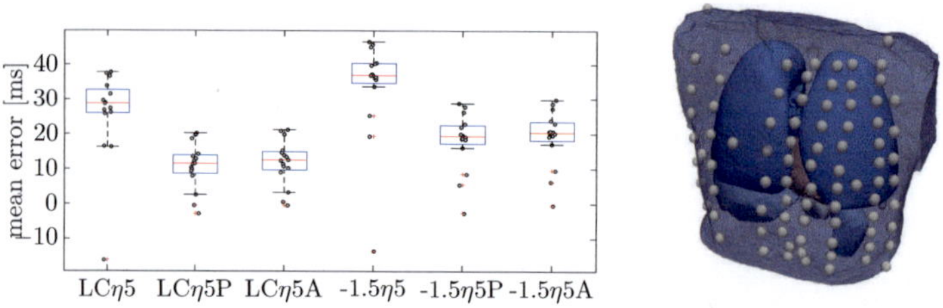

Figure 7.38: Results for Patient 14 (FEM-model), imaging of activation times with and without knowledge from measurements, error with respect to measured LATs (mean [ms]). Bullets represent single PVC beats (n=16). P: a-priori knowledge from 14 ($\approx 25\%$) of the 33 available measurements (built from 42 CARTO LATs), A: all available measurements used as a-priori knowledge.

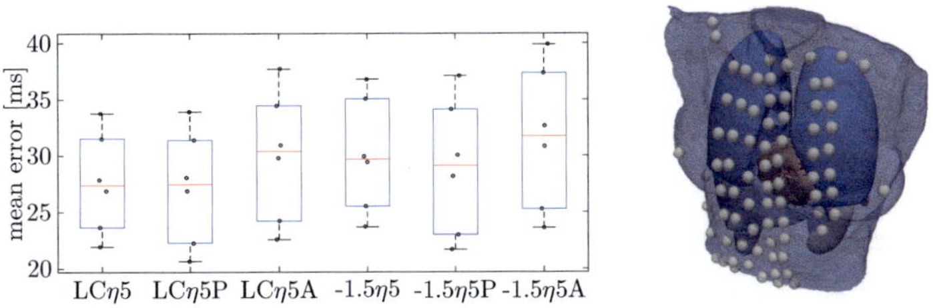

Figure 7.39: Results for Patient 17 (FEM-model), imaging of activation times with and without knowledge from measurements, error with respect to measured LATs (mean [ms]). Bullets represent single PVC beats (n=6). P: a-priori knowledge from 6 ($\approx$ 25%) of the 12 available measurements (built from 16 CARTO LATs), A: all available measurements used as a-priori knowledge.

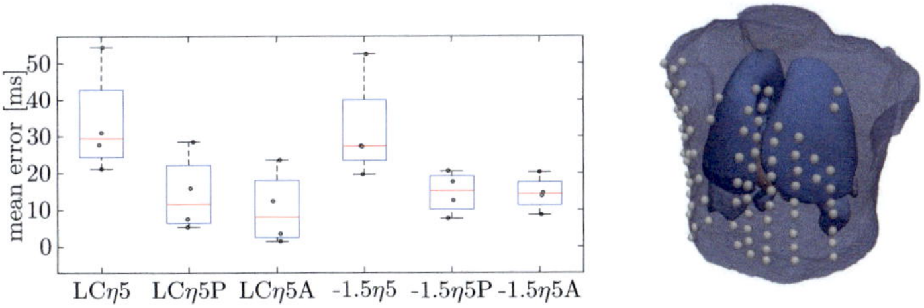

Figure 7.40: Results for Patient 19 (FEM-model), imaging of activation times with and without knowledge from measurements, error with respect to measured LATs (mean [ms]). Bullets represent single PVC beats (n=4). P: a-priori knowledge from 7 ($\approx$ 25%) of the 14 available measurements (built from 24 CARTO LATs), A: all available measurements used as a-priori knowledge.

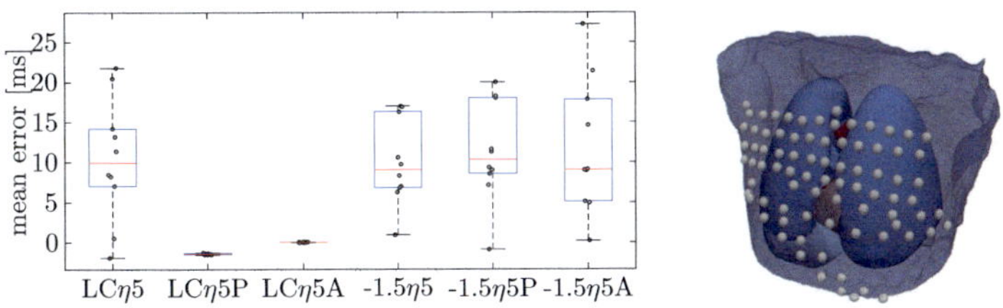

Figure 7.41: Results for Patient 20 (FEM-model), imaging of activation times with and without knowledge from measurements, error with respect to measured LATs (mean [ms]). Bullets represent single PVC beats (n=11). P: a-priori knowledge from 22 ($\approx$ 25%) of the 65 available measurements (built from 88 CARTO LATs), A: all available measurements used as a-priori knowledge.

7.1.4 Tikhonov Spatio-Temporal Method with BSPM Offset Correction

A proof-of-concept study was performed to demonstrate the Tikhonov spatio-temporal method with BSPM offset correction of Sect. 5.4. By the very nature of the method, results are subject to a proper choice of the time points that go into the spatio-temporally regularized window which is used to provide information for the BSPM offset correction: If that window consists only of the time point of evaluation, too much freedom is given to the solver, and the additional degree of freedom in the BSPM is merely allowing the residual error to grow as great as the provided upper limit, i.e., effectively, the offset correction causes the same as a smaller regularization parameter. Therefore, to make the offset correction work properly,

- its upper limit was constrained to 0.1 mV, the lower limit to −0.1 mV.
- a 21 ms window was chosen to provide information for the BSPM offset correction, with the center set at the time of evaluation (OFF), or with that window centered around the R-peak (OFFR).

Results for these approaches are shown in Fig. 7.42 in comparison to the Greensite spatio-temporal method without offset removal (WIN) for the beats (PVCs and effective pacings) of Patient 17 and for a range of regularization parameter values of between 10^{-6} to 10^{-1}. All algorithms use a time window to produce the spatio-temporal regularization, with the time represented by the 6 (p6) or 10 (p10) most relevant temporal singular vectors.

The study shows that results with offset removal and the window around that time of evaluation were worse than those without offset removal. When centering the window around the R-peak (where results are known to be good in ECGI), while evaluating the solution at the R-20 time, results improved (OFFRp10). Studies on further data - and probably also on the parameterization - are required for proper evaluation of the method.

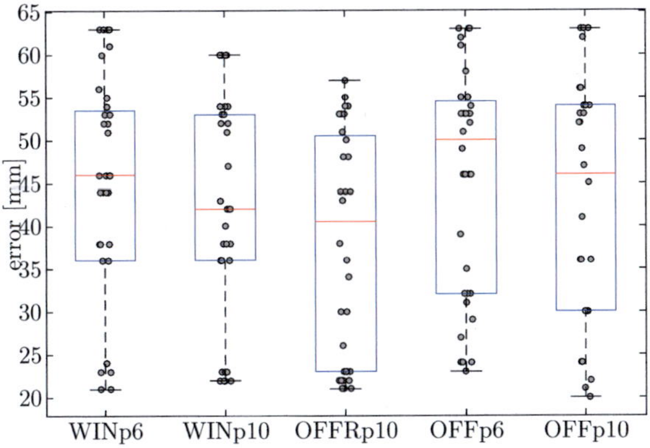

Figure 7.42: BSPM offset correction: localization error for all beats (PVCs and effective pacings, BEM model) of Patient 17 and for a range of regularization parameter values of between 10^{-6} to 10^{-1}. Greensite spatio-temporal method without offset removal (WIN), with offset removal and the window centered at the time of evaluation (OFF), with offset removal and the window centered at the R-peak (OFFR, maximum absolute value of all BSPM signals). The time windows are represented by the 6 (p6) or 10 (p10) first temporal singular vectors.

7.1.5 Solvers with Constraints on the Solution Range

Methods that impose physiological constraints on the solution range of inverse solvers have led to significant advances in simulation studies of ECG imaging [12, 89]. Despite their superior performance in simulation studies and presumably due to modeling errors, such solvers performed worse in this study than the standard Tikhonov or Tikhonov-Greensite spatio-temporal approaches, see Fig. 7.43. Unlike in the previous statistical studies, both solvers were only tested on a single beat of one of the best cases in the study (Patient 17), however across a range of different regularization parameters, with only the best results being presented. In contrary to tests on the quantitative performance, this allows for a qualitative study of the effects that result from the constraints.

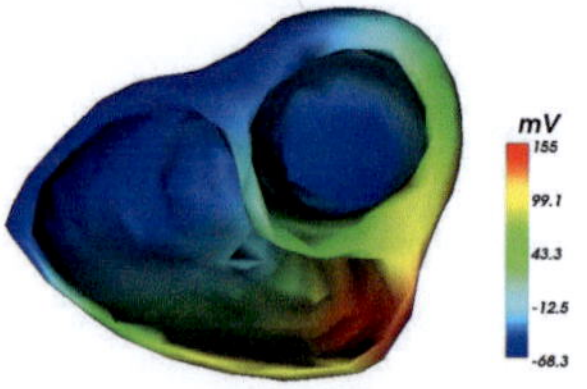

(a) Tikhonov 2nd-order

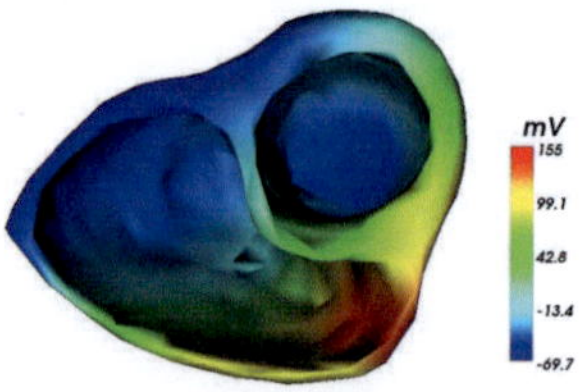

(b) Tikhonov-Greensite

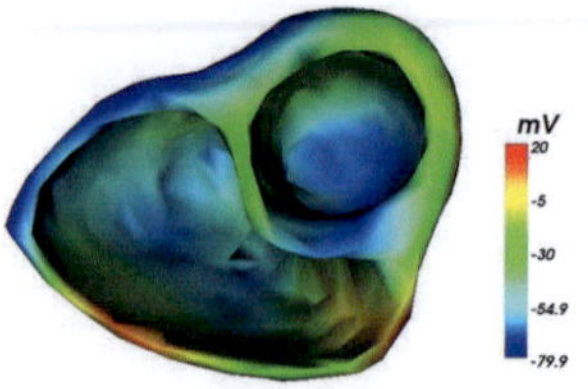

(c) Tikhonov, constraints

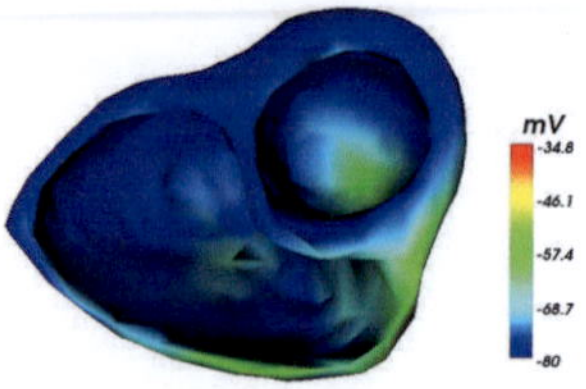

(d) TMV/EP simultaneously

Figure 7.43: Performance of different methods for ECG imaging of TMVs on a PVC beat in Patient 17: (a) Tikhonov 2nd-order [11, 29], (b) Tikhonov-Greensite [96], (c) Tikhonov 2nd-order with constraints on the solution range [89], (d) method for simultaneous reconstruction of TMVs and epicardial potentials (EPs) [12]. For each method, solutions are shown for the best-performing among the tested regularization parameters.

7.2 Validation Study: Ventricular Tachycardia

Cases of induced ventricular tachycardia (VT) were collected at King's College London (KCL) during a procedure that was intended for risk stratification in a decision on whether to implant an implantable cardioverter defibrillator (ICD). Studies were conducted in close cooperation with Kawal Rhode, Aldo Rinaldi and Zhong Chen of KCL, Jatin Relan of INRIA and Martin Krüger of KIT and followed the Wellens 12 stage VT stimulation protocol, which is used in the attempt to induce VT. Due to the nature of the arrhythmia, which must only sustain for a short time, the EnSite non-contact mapping system was used to collect electroanatomical data. Results in this work are shown for Patient 2, who had induced sustained monomorphic VT and was also presented in [137]. Further data studies were conducted within the scope of the project: Patient 01 was originally scheduled for a VT stim study that had to be cancelled, Patient 03 was a test case, Patient 05 had induced sustained monomorphic VT (and had to be cardioverted), in Patient 10 VT was not successfully induced.
Activation sequences (TMVs) of the sustained VT were imaged with the Tikhonov-Greensite spatio-temporal smoothing method (TikhGS, Sect. 4.3.2, L-curve, with the ECG reduced to its 10 most relevant temporal singular vectors). As information on scar locations was known from segmentations of delayed enhancement MRI by KCL, it was studied how the solution is affected when nodes of scar and grey zone are excluded from the solution domain (EXCL). To this end, the respective rows and columns of the lead field matrix and the Laplace operator were removed and the problem was solved with the TikhGS method as before. Scar segmentations were available with separate classes for grey zone and scar, both of which were excluded from the solution domain, and potential boundary conditions or conductivity changes in areas of scar were neglected in the forward model.
Results for the activation sequence are shown in Fig. 7.45 for the TikhGS method, with the activation front popping up in the LV lateral wall after 392 ms, which corresponds to the beginning of the second VT beat in

Fig. 7.44. Similar results are obtained with the EXCL method, where the wavefront is more focused, see Fig. 7.46.

From the imaged TMV activation sequences activation times were computed. To this end, the following procedure was pursued:

- It is analyzed for each node in the heart whether its TMV goes below −40 mV in the time between the end of the previous beat (271 ms) and the end of the overall ECG sequence.
- If this has happened, the next time for the beat to go across 0 mV is sought and referred to the time of the presumed exit point at 392 ms to obtain an activation time.

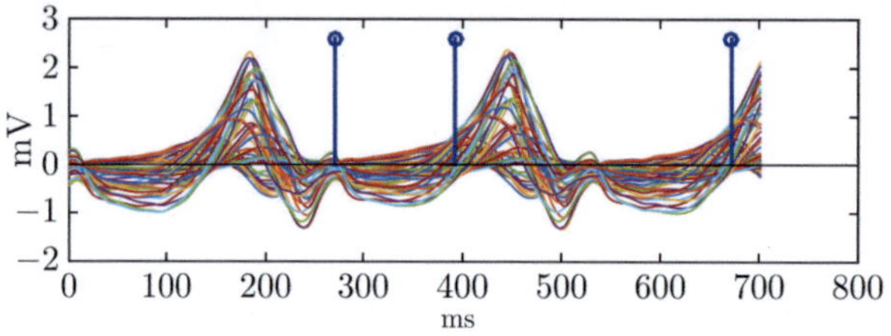

Figure 7.44: BSPM of sustained VT, Patient 02. Three "beats" have been annotated in the excerpt at 148 ms, 380 ms and another one starting at 650 ms, the second of which is evaluated.

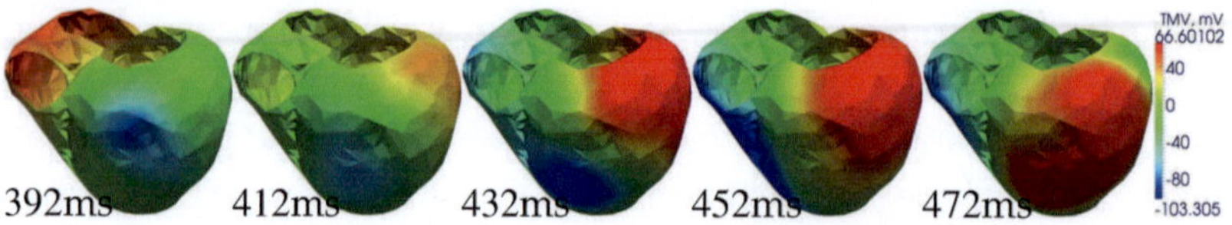

Figure 7.45: Activation sequence (TMVs) of the sustained VT, imaged with the Tikhonov-Greensite spatio-temporal smoothing method (TikhGS), $\lambda = \lambda(\text{L-curve})$, $ECG_{max} = 10$.

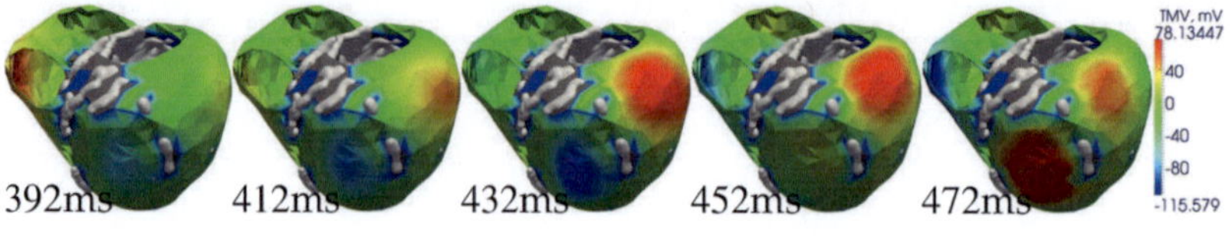

Figure 7.46: Activation sequence (TMVs) of the sustained VT, with nodes of scar and grey zone excluded from the solution domain (EXCL), $\lambda = \lambda(\text{L-curve})$, $ECG_{max} = 10$.

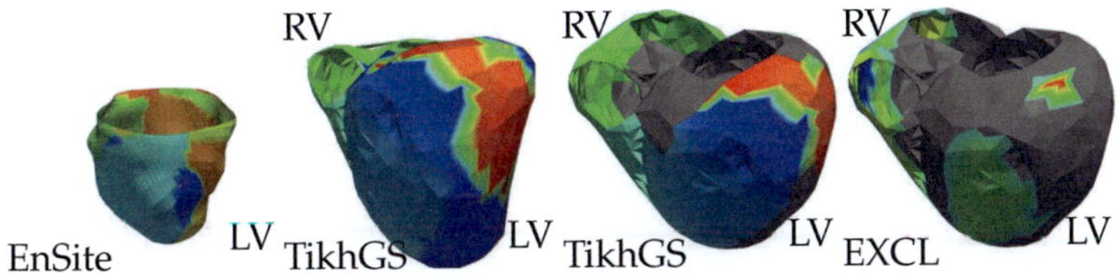

Figure 7.47: Activation times from analysis of the reconstructed TMVs. Right-to-left: activation times computed for the EXCL and the TikhGS method. Two figures on the left: results for TikhGS are rotated for comparison with activation times from the EnSite system. Dark grey: NaN (no activation time computed according to the procedure).

- Nodes that do not go below −40 mV in that interval or that went below but did not thereupon cross 0 mV are flagged as NaN.

These activation times are presented in Fig. 7.47 and compared with the activation sequence from the EnSite measurements of the left ventricle (LV). Early activation times are displayed in blue, late activation times in red (note that this is opposed to the scale that is habitually used in the clinic). Areas with unidentified activation times show up in dark grey. While the activation time map from the EXCL method does obviously not cover much of the activation sequence, it is noteworthy that for the TikhGS method, these areas correspond very well with the scar and grey zone areas found in the delayed enhancement MRI — despite the TikhGS not having any a-priori knowledge on their location. This is demonstrated in detail in Fig. 7.48. This figure shows only the valid activation times; where no activation time could be computed (NaN) only the contours of the ventricles are shown. The display of scar tissue is the switched on (top) and off (bottom). Areas of scar tissue are displayed in dark grey, areas of grey zone in light grey. When looking at the ventricles from both an anterior (left) and a posterior view (right), it is revealed that areas with unidentified activation times (NaN) correspond clearly with the areas where scar tissue was present. As action potentials in areas of scar tissue are known to produce smaller upstrokes than in the normal tissue, this demonstrates clearly the validity of the results.

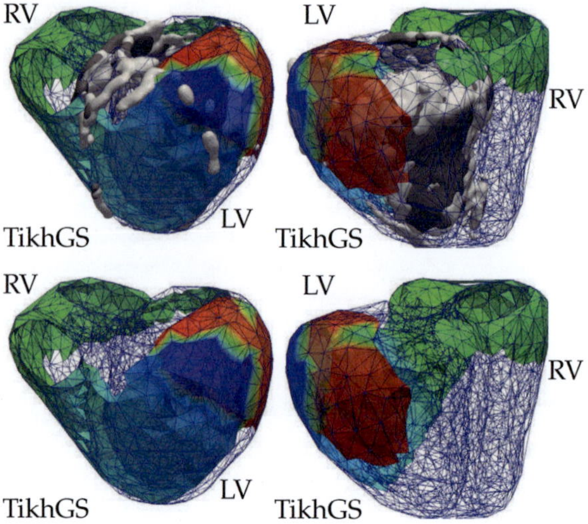

Figure 7.48: Activation times for the Greensite method with all nodes included in the solution domain (Fig. 7.45). Scar tissue from delayed enhancement MRI is displayed in dark grey and grey zone in light grey. Upper figures: MRI scar data depicted in grey, lower figures: MRI scar data switched off.

7.2.1 BSPM Smoothness Based Baseline Correction

The VT activation time imaging study was repeated with the BSPM baseline corrected as proposed in Eq. 6.10-Eq. 6.12. The method optimizes the BSPM's spatial smoothness, i.e., close channels may not differ significantly, while also minimizing the energy of the resulting BSPM. This is achieved by tuning only the BSPM offset, assuming it is the same for all time steps. Results are shown in Fig. 7.49 (BSPM after smoothness based baseline correction) and Fig. 7.50 (baseline correction performed by the algorithm). For comparison, ECG imaging with the TikhGS method was performed with a predefined regularization parameter ($\lambda = 5 \cdot 10^{-5}$), and results were produced before (lower row) and after BSPM correction (upper row), see Fig. 7.51. Activation sequences differ only slightly, despite significant corrections being made, see Fig. 7.50.

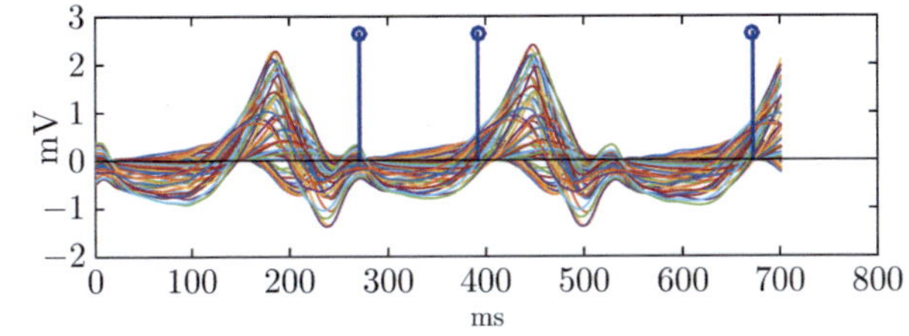

Figure 7.49: BSPM of sustained VT from Fig. 7.44 after smoothness based baseline correction.

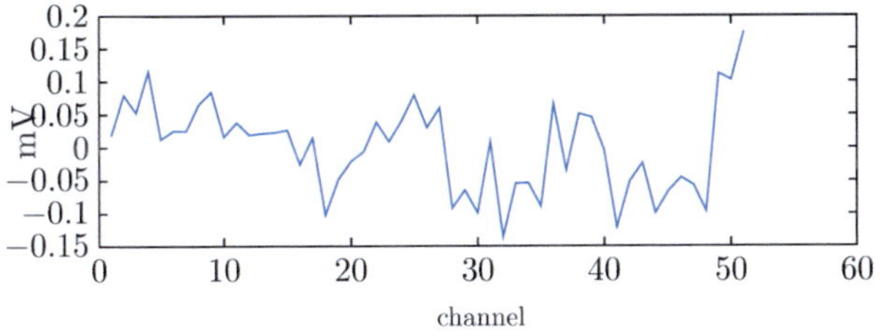

Figure 7.50: Baseline correction performed on the BSPM in Fig. 7.44.

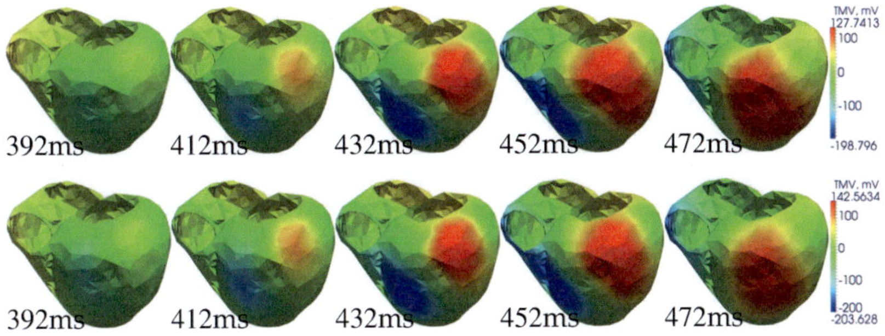

Figure 7.51: Results with the smoothness based baseline correction (upper row). Lower row: results before baseline correction. Activation sequence (TMVs) of the sustained VT, imaged with the Tikhonov-Greensite spatio-temporal smoothing method (TikhGS), $\lambda = 5 \cdot 10^{-5}$, $ECG_{max} = 10$.

Part IV

Discussion

8

Discussion and Conclusions

Two validation studies of ECG imaging were performed within the scope of this work, and some new methods for ECG imaging proposed. For the validation studies, this section will discuss the results in the context of previous works, discuss modeling errors (and for the PVC study also the censoring and time of evaluation), to finally conclude with recommendations. For the proposed methods, it will discuss the results and potential of each method individually.

8.1 Validation Study: Premature Ventricular Contractions

In the clinical validation study with UMM, altogether 201 pacings and 75 PVC beats were manually annotated, linked to their validation data and evaluated with the most established ECG imaging methods available in our group, with models based on both the boundary element method and the finite element method. These results were presented as statistics that include all annotated beats as in [65].

8.1.1 Censoring and Time of Evaluation

The best time of evaluation was found to be surprisingly late, and the censoring of beats was surprisingly ineffective:

- For the imaging of excitation origins (Sect. 7.1.2 on page 91), among various schemes for the time of evaluation, the best results were obtained with the R-20 scheme, which is to pick the BSPM signal at 20% of the QRS length before the R-peak. It was subsequently used for all methods in the study, apart from those that produce activation times from the entire QRS. Although this is the latest of all tested times of evaluation, which reflects an excitation spread that has propagated significantly from its origin, it produces the results with best localization accuracy, owing supposedly to the better signal-to-noise ratio at these times and to the solvers being better suited to less focused and hence smoother solutions.
- A censoring of beats has been proposed to identify beats with unusually large signal at the QRS end, presumably reflecting baseline wander in the BSPM or floating electrode channels. It was initially

used for the BEM models but then dropped, as results for censored beats had rather small localization errors. I.e., results clearly contradict the premise that great signal at the QRS end correlates with bad ECG imaging solutions. At first, this is an unexpected result. But it reflects three things: first, beats were annotated manually and carefully selected to have little baseline wander; second: electrode channels with floating signal had already been carefully identified and removed - although they pop up for some beats during the experiments; third: beats with great signal at the QRS end might actually be caused by the ablations taking place during the experiment, leading to a change of conduction patterns and scar-related ST-elevation. The latter might also explain the change in the PVC beat morphology during the run of the study in Fig. 6.9 and Fig. 6.10 on page 77, which served as the initial motivation for the censoring.

BEM models

The following results were obtained for the study for localization of excitation origins with BEM models that include the endocardial and epicardial surface.

- Comparison of methods: for BEM models, while the Tikhonov-based methods without knowledge from simulations (Tikh, TikhGS, AT-intT2) produced large localization errors, results with the different maximum a posteriori (MAP) approaches and the critical times approach (CritTeff35) delivered relatively similar results for paced beats in the order of 25 mm median error, but also for PVC beats with 20 to 30 mm error, see Fig. 7.7 and Fig. 7.6 on page 95. Among the best methods, the localization error was clearly governed by the choice of patient, rather than the imaging method. For this reason, it may be concluded that the greatest portion of the error is a result of modeling errors rather than errors caused by the nature of the inverse solvers (although it also depends on the origins of the beats, which is obviously different for different patients, see below). The performance of the solvers may rather be reflected in the median localization error of the best patient, which for effective pacings in Fig. 7.7 on page 96 lay in the range of ≈ 10 mm, with the MAP method delivering again the best results.

- Results with the best method (BEM models): For the MAP method, the following findings were made (Patient 06 is excluded from evaluation, as it has only seven ECG channels available):
  - Results for different patients, including statistics on the localization error for excitation origins in different areas of the heart (see Sect. 7.1.2):
    - For Patient 11, localization errors were large for all measured events (mean errors were $\in [29,62]$ mm). With large errors in many different areas of the heart, this is presumably due to the patient model.
    - Patients 12 and 19 may or may not be a bad model: mean localization errors are large ($\in [20,50]$ mm and $\in [38,52]$ mm), but all excitations originate from the septum (despite some single lateral beats in Patient 19 which were also localized with large error).
    - Patient 09 shows very well the effect of non-unique solutions in ECG imaging. As in Fig. 4.2b on page 27, despite the effective beat EFFx27 being imaged very well at 3 mm error, the PVC, which is in the septum, is imaged at 44 mm mean error.
    - Mean errors for Patient 20 are large ($\in [17,42]$ mm) except for the PVC (< 20 mm, which is < 10 mm from the minimum distance to the validation), which is despite the patient being among the two best models according to Tab. 7.1. Still and due to the results for the PVC, it can be assumed to be a good model in general: the large errors can be linked to most of the excitation origins being at the level of the valve. The Patient may hence profit from a more inclusive segmentation of the ventricles in that area.
    - Patient 17 has very good results (error < 20 mm for all beats, < 15 mm for most effective beats, except for one single outlier that leads to a misleading mean error range of 5 to 40 mm). Another good model is that of Patient 14, which has errors mostly < 20 mm for the PVC and EFFx57 and is also among the

two best models according to the quality of the processing in Tab. 7.1. It shows again clearly the effect of non-unique solutions in that some distant outliers exist in the statistics of EFFx57, and in that localization errors vary strongly for some of the beats, despite being from the exact same area.

- For Patient 13 some good results were generated (errors for the PVC are mostly < 20 mm). Yet, a broad spectrum of errors exists for the effective beats EFF, with strong variation despite excitation origins being from the same area, and the range of mean errors is 14 mm to 27 mm. These errors may be due to inaccuracies in the models that have dynamic behaviour, such as breathing-related effects. With the area of excitation origins not being exactly in the middle of the septum, it would also be interesting to study with the method proposed in [23] if it is still affected from having non-unique BSPMs.

– Excitation spread over time (at the time of evaluation, 10ms before and after): For the best beats, the excitation spread is physiologically reasonable for Patients 09, 11, 13, 14, 17, 19 and 20. However, with limitations for Patients 09, 13, 14 and 20: The imaged origin is shifted from the septal origin in case of the PVC in Patient 09; the first shown time instances in Patients 14 and 20 appear to have noise-induced artifacts, and while the second shown time instance in Patient 13 is unreasonable. For Patient 12, the excitation spreads show little dynamics and start from the lateral wall opposite the origin, which is at the septum. This demonstrates that the best localization errors with the MAP method were not achieved with artifacts (e.g. from baseline wander, that could as well lead to good solutions by chance) but with solutions that represent physiologically propagating TMVs.

To summarize, while Patient 11 seems to have large modeling errors, Patients 09, 14, 17 and potentially also Patient 12 and 19 seem to have little, and results may strongly profit from inverse solvers that manage to deal better with the underdeterminedness of the problem. While data in Patient 13 suffers from regional-independent variations that are presumably due to dynamic modeling errors such as breathing effects, results for Patient 20 suffer from the excitation events being at the level of the valve, which is not included in the model. Best results were not based on artifacts, but represent physiologically propagating TMVs.

FEM models

The following paragraph will discuss the results for localization of excitation origins with FEM models.

- Results for methods MAP and ATintT2 with respect to the BEM models: While results with the MAP method had been best in case of the BEM models, they performed worse with the FEM model. Errors increase by $> 1\,\text{cm}$ for the PVCs and by $> 0.5\,\text{cm}$ for the effective pacings. On the other hand, results with the ATintT2 method improved by $1\,\text{cm}$ for PVCs and by $< 1.5\,\text{cm}$ for effective pacings. This may either be due to the increased ill-posedness (in terms of non-uniqueness of the solutions) when imaging transmural TMVs compared to surface TMVs, but it is more likely due to the (rather simple) model that was used for training the covariance matrix in the MAP method, which is probably less suited for volumetric meshes. As the ATintT2 method produces great errors for both kinds of models, it should be studied whether the L-curve method is choosing the regularization parameter from an appropriate range. Further, it should be studied whether the ideal choice for the QRS interval has been made - regardless of the underlying volume conductor discretization method.
- Choice of the best method, interpretation in context of results with the BEM models: Best results were achieved with the MODcct method, i.e. with a simple model of the cardiac excitation spread, where solutions are judged by their correlation with the BSPM in time. Since it takes into account the entire excitation spread of the QRS, results with the method are expected to be superior to the results with the MAP method and the BEM models especially in case of excitation origins in areas that often have non-unique solutions (i.e., the septum). On the other hand, results are expected to be worse in general in areas where the coarse heart mesh does not represent the cardiac anatomy

very well, i.e., especially where excitation bridges are not represented in the model (i.e., presumably at the base and close to the valves).

- Results with the best method (FEM models): For the MODcct method, the following findings were made, see Sect. 7.1.2. Patient 06 is excluded from evaluation, as it has only seven ECG channels available.
  - For Patient 09, results were indeed slightly better for beats at the septum and the beats that had previously been missed with the BEM models. The results for the best beats with the BEM approach, however, could not be obtained with the FEM model.
  - For Patient 11, results have improved a lot for both the PVC (error $< 10\,\text{mm}$) and the effective beats EFFx47 and EFFx64 ($\approx 10\,\text{mm}$), which renders Patient 11 one of the best models. I.e., either the method of solving the inverse problem or the representation of Patient 11 with surface meshes has caused a significant improvement of results (errors with BEM were around 30 to 40 mm).
  - For Patient 12, results were relatively similar to those with the BEM method, revealing that even the chosen model-based approach cannot correctly localize excitation origins in the septum.
  - For Patient 13, results were slightly worse for the PVC, compared to the BEM approach, but slightly better and much more stable for the effective pacings. This is despite all origins being in the area of the outflow tract.
  - For Patient 14, results were worse by $\approx 1\,\text{cm}$, yet again more stable compared to the BEM-based results.
  - For Patient 17, results were very similar to those with the BEM models.
  - For Patient 19, results were worse for the PVC and better for effective beat EFFx52, compared to those with the BEM method.
  - For Patient 20, results were much better with the MODcct and the FEM model and slightly worse and again more stable for the effective beats. The localization error for the PVC here was smaller than the origin's distance to the nearest point in the mesh. This is due to the excitation origin having been identified in the solution as a mean position, which may have lain in the lumen under certain conditions.

To conclude, localization errors were usually worse, yet also more stable than for the MAP method and the BEM models. The notion that a model-based approach would deal better with excitation origins in the septum could not be supported with findings, neither the notion that it would work worse in areas close to the valves. Patient 11 who had bad results with the BEM method and was considered to have great modeling error to that end is now found to produce very good results, contradicting that assumption. Note though that models had been smoothed and simplified for the BEM models, which may also explain the changes as resulting from errors in the cardiac or thoracic anatomy. Also, the finding that modeling errors for Patient 13 originate from dynamic effects could be contradicted by the finding that for FEM models, results have little variation at relatively good quality.

BEM models: averaging of multiple beats

For the BEM models and the MAP method, it was tested whether results improved when averaging multiple beats of the same cardiac event. Results turned out differently than expected. In contrary to the hypothesis that noise on the beats would be Gaussian, the averaging of multiple beats should have improved signal quality. However, results did not improve and even worsened to some degree. This may be interpreted in two ways: either the noise was not Gaussian as assumed and errors such as baseline wander in single beats have dominated the noise reduction, or the beats themselves were not classified well enough for consideration in the averaging (in the study, all beats of the same annotated event were averaged).

FEM models: imaging of activation times

The imaging of activation times with the proposed framework that facilitates the use of a-priori knowledge from measured local activation times has demonstrated the functioning of the method. Even more importantly, it has demonstrated the limitations of the quality measure used in this study, as even with all LAT measurements available, the activation origin was not accurately localized. Validation measurements should therefore be evaluated statistically in the future to mark excitation origins rather than picking single points with the earliest activation times — or single ablation points.

8.1.2 Comparison with Results of Other Groups

As shown in Tab. 4.2, which describes the state-of-the-art in ECG imaging validation studies according to literature, most validation studies have been performed for the reconstruction of epicardial potentials and only few for the imaging of epi- and endocardial potentials. These few studies can be grouped with the surface activation time studies of Tilg et al. which also imaged the endo- and epicardium at the same time. This work falls under the latter categories for the results with the BEM models, as these include endo- and epicardial surfaces as well — yet with the difference of imaging TMVs as sources. Validation for TMVs is practically only possible for their activation times or imaged excitation origins, i.e., the work of Tilg et al. [68, 74–76] serve as adequate reference, where only [74] deals with ventricular excitation, along with that of Erem et al. [65].

The localization errors for imaging of focal excitation origins are greater than the errors found in the previous studies by Tilg et al., where pacing origins in the atria were imaged at 6 to 14 mm accuracy. Errors are also greater than in the study of localizing excitation origins from WPW pathways, which result in a ventricular phenomenon and had been imaged at 19 mm accuracy. This may either be due to the BEM models being better suited for atrial signals, or to the fact that Tilg et al. have included the lungs in their models, while the present models only had the heart modeled. Yet, the results of this work are in the range of the mean errors of (3 to 5 cm) reported for the ventricles in [65] and [73], where the localization error was 13 – 28 mm and increased significantly to 28 – 67 mm in the presence of scar. It cannot be concluded whether the differences in results with respect to the atria, and also the ventricles in a presumably healthy-substrate-case, stem from any particular errors. For that reason, an analysis of the modeling errors is made in the following, and conclusions are drawn on how models can be approved

— keeping in mind the errors revealed for the origins in the septum, which rather suggest improvements in the inverse solvers.

8.1.3 Modeling Errors

Apart from their sensitivity to noise in the BSPM, solutions of the inverse problem are strongly affected by modeling errors in A. As summarized in [11, Sect. 4.8] and studied in silico in [38, 173], multiple sources of modeling errors exist that originate from the fusion of the imaging and measurement modalities as well as the inaccuracy or limited applicability of the individual methods (methods for model creation are presented in Sect. 6).

The following modeling steps were performed in the validation studies of this work and are hence discussed regarding the sources of modeling error:

- Anatomical modeling and parameterization of tissue conductivities
  - Errors of MRI co-registration have been computed and objectively evaluated, see Tab. 7.1 and Sect. B in the Appendix. Apart from Patient 19, for which the heart model was obtained from an actual 3-D scan, cine MRI data was used for all patients in the PVC study. These models bear a great risk of introducing relevant modeling error, as interpolation of the data had to be performed between the imaged layers. The data also did not allow for a segmentation of the atrial blood, and the layer of the atrio-ventricular valves and the position of the valves in the outflow tracts could only approximately be identified, despite being the area of excitation origin in many of the cases. The use of cine MRI, however, is in line with the proposed methods from previous validation studies of ECGI [155] and seems to be the only choice for radiation-free imaging in the presence of frequent ventricular arrhythmia. For the VT stim cases, a 3-D navigated whole heart scan was used, together with an automatic model-based segmentation procedure, leading to way superior heart models.

  - Though studies exist that prove the importance of accurate models [174], the best choice of organs to be segmented for ECGI is an open question, as other groups argue against the importance of complex models [175]. Additional segmentations improve the anatomical representation, but may also induce error in case of erroneous segmentations and, more importantly, in the case of inaccurate conductivities being assigned to the tissue. This is coupled with the effect of cardiac signals being attenuated in their BSPM representation, which makes ECG imaging possible to only a certain degree of accuracy — and might influence strongly-regularized solutions less than inverse solutions with greater degree of freedom. Also, too many surfaces can lead to numerical problems in BEM forward calculations. Two orthogonal approaches were followed in this work: for the FEM-models, multiple organs and tissue structures were segmented and assigned conductivity values from literature (however, we could not model the atria due to the quality of MR images in the presence of arrhythmia). For BEM-models, only the thorax and heart surface were modeled, again with values from literature. Based on [176], an approach has been developed within the scope of this work to parameterize tissue conductivities from BSPM measurements of few effective pacings of the myocardium. Also, it could be shown theoretically that lead field matrices can be parameterized immediately without expensive calculations on-site in the catheter laboratory [177]. Such a technique may benefit the quality of both BEM or FEM models significantly in the future.
- Cardiac anisotropy
  - According to a simulation study in [178], the anisotropy of cardiac fiber orientation and hence conductivity is negligible for the inverse solvers used by the group. The study compares solutions of the inverse problem with the boundary element method for BSPMs from FEM forward calculations that take cardiac anisotropy into account. Nevertheless, our group intends to use transmembrane voltages as the source model in ECG imaging, which for correct

transmural results requires information on fiber orientation. Also, it has been demonstrated that fiber orientation may be derived from diffusion-tensor MRI [179] and has great impact on simulations of cardiac excitation propagation [180]. Hence, it is believed that with rule-based cardiac fiber anisotropy introduced in the ventricles [104, 140], forward calculations become more precise also for patient data, especially in case it can be measured in-vivo [181] in the future. Still, studies for both hypotheses are conducted in this work, as both FEM and BEM models are used. Rule-based anisotropy information is included in the former, but not in the latter.

- Respiration
  - The effect of respiration on results in ECGI was found to have significant impact on the correlation coefficient of inverse solutions with the simulations [182]. Cardiac MR scans and thorax scans were therefore recorded in this work during breath-hold, which is in line with the recommended procedure for ECGI studies [155]. Also, it was ensured that MRI scans were taken in end-expiration, not inspiration, to being close to the realistic level during normal breathing. Still, respiratory levels were not recorded, which may explain the different results for different beats of the same event in the PVC study.
- Heart motion
  - Cardiac motion was not modeled in the present studies. However, it was ensured that recordings across all recordings were taken in end-diastolic phase. Using a static heart anatomy was shown in [183] to have little impact on the depolarization phase of the heart, while having strong effects on the T-wave. All signals in this work, apart from the VT study, have been evaluated during QRS only. For studies on the effect of heat motion on ECGI, see also [184, 185].
- Mesh quality
  - The ideal resolution of FEM meshes for forward calculations was studied within the scope of this work [26] and applied according

to the findings. However, similar studies were not performed for the resolution of coarse meshes that represent the solution of the inverse problem in the FEM models. Still, by using BEM models as well, with the meshes smoothed and reduced in complexity, it may be claimed that again, a very different and hence orthogonal approach has been tested on the data.

- Electrode localization
  - For electrode localization, according to [113–115], displacement errors of 1 to 2 mm may be tolerated in ECG imaging. However, other studies have shown that errors of 5 mm [38, Sect. 8.1] or 7 mm [116, Sect. 7.3] may lead to significantly worse results. To ensure good-enough accuracy of the electrode localization, a system for electrode localization was developed within the scope of this work with 1 ± 1 mm accuracy.
- BSPM processing and annotation
  - Great efforts were made to use the best possible BSPM processing method, as it has great impact on the ECG imaging solution, especially for solvers without spatio-temporal regularization schemes. Initially, different filters were tested with different cut-off frequencies and characteristics. Also, different approaches have been studied for removal of the BSPM offset, and new methods have been proposed for its identification. Also averaging of multiple beats was tested, and annotations of the beats in the studies were meticulously checked.

8.1.4 Conclusion

To conclude, all steps in the modeling pipeline have been optimized, apart from

- cardiac imaging for model generation (advances have only been made towards the very end of the study)
- the resolution of the coarse geometry for FEM models
- the representation of cardiac anisotropy in lead the field matrix of the FEM models

Also, in future studies, it should be taken care of the patients being imaged with MRI while not showing arrhythmic activity, which will strongly improve the quality of heart models. Otherwise, studies should only be planned if MRI protocols for arrhythmia detection are available. Further, to reduce modeling error, BSPM measurements should be done on the MRI table, and the electrodes should be directly marked in the MRI images. This would reduce co-registration errors and is typically done in commercial applications of ECG imaging. On the other hand, if measurements are done in the catheter lab, BSPM beats can be linked directly to the synchronously recorded cardiac activity, which facilitates the imaging of non-repeating cardiac events such as pacings. The latter may be used to improve models in the future — and single measurements of cardiac electrograms may be used in the future to improve results in ECG imaging. The datasets of this study are suited to validate such methods, and the proposed camera system may be used by groups in the field to localize electrodes in a catheter lab setting for future studies.

8.2 Validation Study: Ventricular Tachycardia

Localizing origins of ventricular tachycardia for treatment in radio-frequency ablation therapy is a great clinical challenge for conventional non-invasive methods [70]. To the knowledge of the author, several groups have performed animal studies on ECG imaging of VT [114, 186], but only two papers describe a validation of the method in human [66, 73], apart from a case study in magnetocardiography [187]. In [66] nine patients were imaged during sustained VT, and ECG imaging results of the epicardium were compared with electroanatomical maps of the endocardium (see limitations in [66]). In [73], no activation sequences were recorded. The present study is presumably the first to image VT as transmural distribution of TMVs, i.e. with volumetric models. These models and the use of TMVs allowed for an introduction of scar information in the solution. Results demonstrate that the applied algorithms are able to image activation patterns and the excitation origin with good accuracy. Also, even without introducing information of the cardiac scar location, areas of scar were clearly visible in the ECG imaging results as areas where activation times were not computed for little signal activity in the TMVs. Results are therefore concluded to represent well the excitation pattern in the ventricles and shall be evaluated quantitatively in the future to support the qualitative finding. For the VT study, from the point of modeling quality, it is important to note that the models of the VT study have the best possible accuracy, with perfectly imaged thoraxes that were automatically taken at the same breathing level as the navigated heart scans, and with automatic model-based segmentation tools being used to build highly accurate models of the whole heart, including (manual) segmentations of scar tissue. Also, according to [50, Sect. 9.7.3.2], validation measurements with the EnSite system have been shown to have good accuracy within 40 mm of the catheter [188], i.e. within the range where results have been evaluated in the present study.

8.3 Proposed Methods

Within the scope of the validation studies and in the context of previous simulation studies, the following methods have been proposed:

- A framework to enhance ECG imaging solutions with single intracardiac measurements during ablation procedures with little arrhythmic activity.
- A spatio-temporal Tikhonov method that identifies the optimal offset in the BSPM.
- A BSPM smoother that identifies its optimal offset through optimization of the smoothness of the BSPM and by minimization of its energy.
- A state-space model for ECG imaging that introduces regularization in the solutions of its measurement-based corrections by augmentation of the measurement signal (not described explicitly in this thesis, see [86])
- A new variant of the critical times method

- A simple model-based ECG imaging approach that performed best for FEM.

Part V

Appendix

A

Effect of mesh resolutions in the forward problem

The effect of resolution parameters for mesh generation with the computational geometry algorithms library (CGAL) [139] was tested in [142] for forward calculations of the electrocardiogram in a simplified thorax model. The study is extended here to cover not only the resolution, but all relevant mesh generation parameters, and it is repeated in a realistic thorax model to study also the parameters that are relevant for the meshing of the thorax and organs.

> Note: All meshing parameters of this study are explained in detail in [142, Tab. 1].

A.1 Simplified Thorax Model

A.1.1 Resolution

A single TMV source is placed in the ventricles to study resolution effects in a simplified thorax model. To explore the limits of resolution effects in the volume of potential cardiac sources, first, the entire

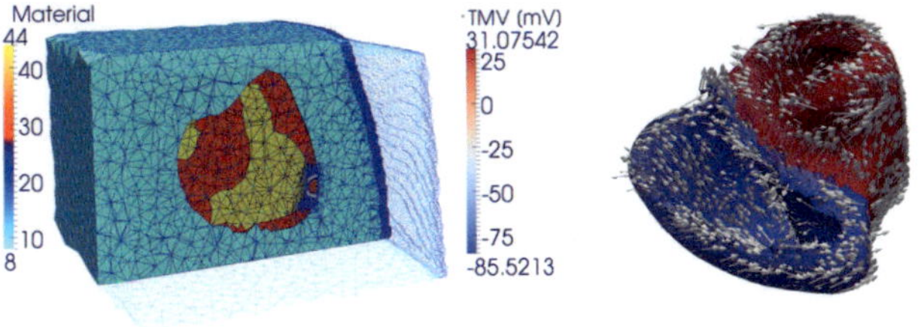

Figure A.1: Left: simplified thorax model and source in study on meshing parameters for forward calculations. Right: rule-based fiber orientation. Patient 19, figures adapted from [142, Fig. 1,3]

heart is refined, for the setup see [142][Fig. 2], and later on, the resolution is only adjusted in a region-of-interest around the actual cardiac source, see Fig. A.1 (left). Fiber orientation according to [140] was produced at 0.4 mm resolution to set the conductivity tensors, see Fig. A.1 (right). With all other mesh generation parameters fixed, parameter refine_cell_size is tuned according to Tab. A.1, where the first range stands for the study with refinement of the entire heart and the second range stands for the study with a refined region-of-interest (ROI).

Parameter	Range
facet_angle (f_a)	25°
facet_size (f_s)	7.5 mm
facet_distance (f_d)	7.5 mm
cell_radius_ edge_ratio (c_r_e)	3
cell_size (c_s)	8 mm
refine_facet_size (r_f_s)	7.5 mm
refine_cell_size (r_c_s)	$[0.55, 0.6, \ldots, 1, 1.5, \ldots, 8]$ mm and $[0.3, 0.35, \ldots, 1, 1.5, \ldots, 8]$ mm

Table A.1: Choice of Parameters: Resolution Study in Simplified Thorax Model

The resulting ECGs for the different resolutions are computed and compared to the ECG with the highest resolution as root mean squared error in Fig. A.2, the respective ECG signals themselves are presented in Fig. A.3 and Fig. A.4.
Results show, as in [142], that the greatest resolution-related effects diminish below a resolution of approximately 5 mm. Below 1 mm, only marginal effects on the computed ECG remain. For further discussion of these effects, see [142].

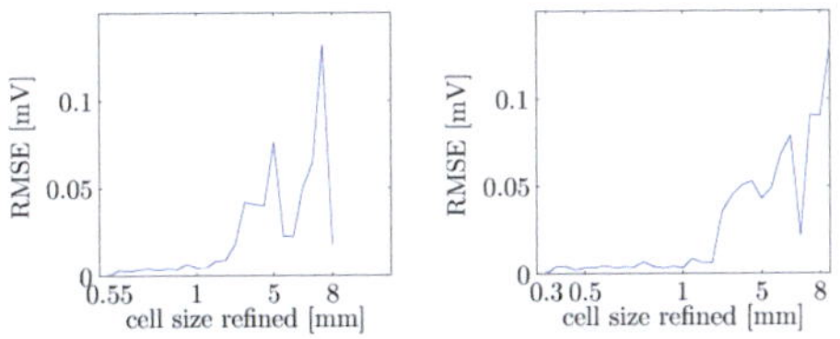

(a) Refined: heart. (b) Refined: ROI.

Figure A.2: Root mean squared error of the computed ECG with respect to the ECG obtained for the highest tested resolution. Left: first setup, the resolution of the cardiac tissue is adjusted for the entire heart. Right: second setup, the resolution is only adjusted in a region-of-interest around the actual cardiac source (results are comparable to those in [142][Fig. 6]).

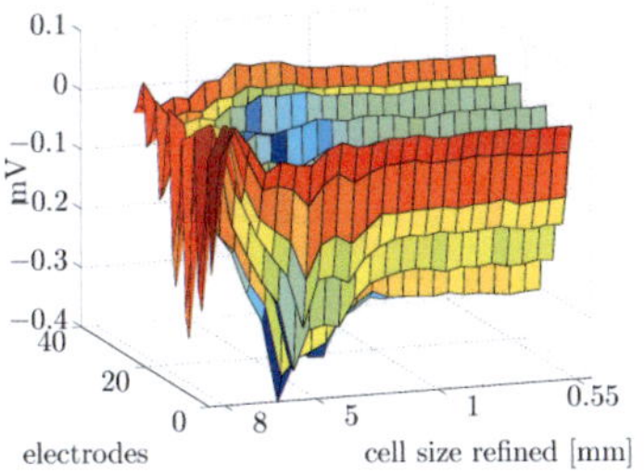

Figure A.3: Refined: heart. The ECG signal is shown for all 28 electrodes over the resolution of the refined cardiac tissue.

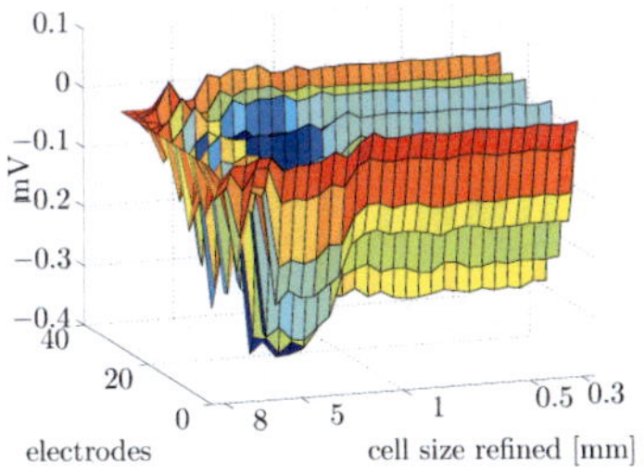

Figure A.4: Refined: ROI. The ECG signal is shown for all 28 electrodes over the resolution of the refined cardiac tissue.

A.1.2 Facet Angle

With the same simplified thorax model and the cardiac tissue refinement already parameterized at 1 mm refinement for the entire heart, the effect of the facet_angle parameter was studied, see parameters in Tab. A.2.

Parameter	Range
facet_angle (f_a)	$[15, 16, \ldots, 34]^\circ$
facet_size (f_s)	7.5 mm
facet_distance (f_d)	7.5 mm
cell_radius_ edge_ratio (c_r_e)	3
cell_size (c_s)	8 mm
refine_facet_size (r_f_s)	7.5 mm
refine_cell_size (r_c_s)	1 mm

Table A.2: Choice of Parameters: Variation of Facet Angle in Simplified Thorax Model

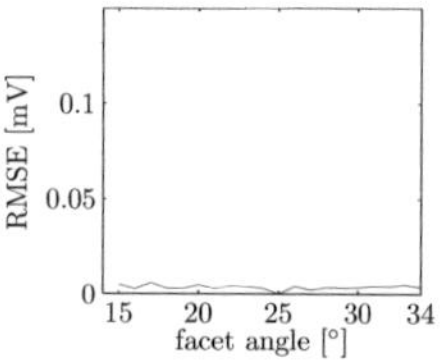

Figure A.5: Root mean squared error of the computed ECG with respect to the ECG obtained for a facet_angle of 25°.

The resulting ECGs for the different facet angles are computed and compared to the ECG resulting from a facet_angle of 25° in Fig. A.5, the respective ECG signals themselves are presented in Fig. A.6.
From the study, it is apparent that using the resolutions found in the previous study, the facet_angle parameter has no significant effect on the ECG. As it has been tested over a reasonable range from small angles to up to 34°, which is beyond the 30° at and below which convergence is guaranteed, and as the mesher crashed for higher angles, it can be concluded that for the given problem and with the resolution parameters used, facet_angle may well be set to 25° in the following steps of this work.

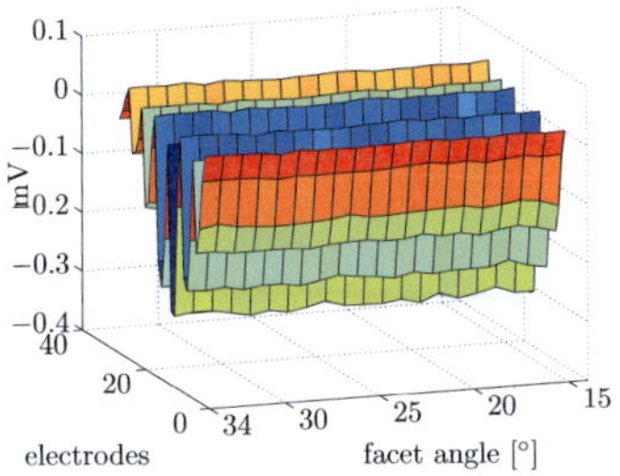

Figure A.6: Refined: heart. The ECG signal is shown for all 28 electrodes over the resolution of the refined cardiac tissue.

A.2 Realistic Thorax Model

With a resolution of 1 mm set for the cardiac tissue and the facet_angle set to 25 °, as the previous studies suggest, meshing parameters for the tissue classes of a realistic thorax model were tested in the following. Meshing parameters facet_size and cell_size were tuned while a specific facet_distance was given, see Fig. A.7. This study was repeated for different facet distances, see Tab. A.3. The cell_size was only reduced down to 3 mm, as forward calculations failed for all attempts with 2 mm. For the realistic thorax model the segmentation of Patient 19 was used, with specific tissue classes assigned to the heart, liver, lungs, kidneys, spleen, aorta, stomach and skeletal muscle, and with 185 electrodes on the thorax surface.

Errors in Fig. A.8, Fig. A.9, Fig. A.10, Fig. A.2 and Fig. A.12 are in general an order of magnitude smaller than in the studies of cardiac tissue refinement in Fig. A.1 or Fig. A.13. Convergence can be seen towards higher resolutions, and errors are greatest for facet and cell sizes > 10 mm. For a facet_distance of 1 mm, errors are greatest for small facet sizes, in contrary to the findings for other facet distances, which may reflect problems with the robustness of the mesh optimization at these levels. To conclude, while no meticulous attention is required for the resolution of the thorax model and its tissue classes in case the resolution of the heart mesh is fine enough, it is still relevant to keep cell sizes and facet sizes below 10 mm. As mesh generation tended to fail in some of the

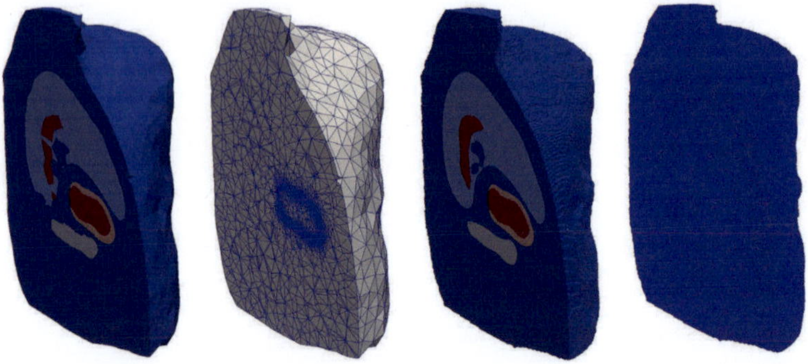

(a) facet_size 20 mm, cell_size 20 mm. (b) Mesh edges in (a). (c) facet_size 1 mm, cell_size 2 mm. (d) Mesh edges in (c).

Figure A.7: Realistic thorax model, facet_distance 16 mm. Material classes are displayed for different resolutions. In a separate image, the surface edges of the respective meshes are displayed in blue over grey.

cases with greater facet_distance than 0.5 mm (results are displayed as zeros for such cases in the graphs), it is further concluded that a small facet_distance tends to guarantee a successful meshing procedure for the setup in the study.

Parameter	Range
facet_angle (f_a)	25°
facet_size (f_s)	[20, 15, 10, 5, 4, . . . , 1] mm
facet_distance (f_d)	[16, 10, 5, 1, 0.5] mm
cell_radius_ edge_ratio (c_r_e)	3
cell_size (c_s)	[20, 15, 10, 5, 4, 3] mm
refine_facet_size (r_f_s)	7.5 mm
refine_cell_size (r_c_s)	1 mm

Table A.3: Choice of Parameters: Variation of Facet Size and Cell Size in Realistic Thorax Model

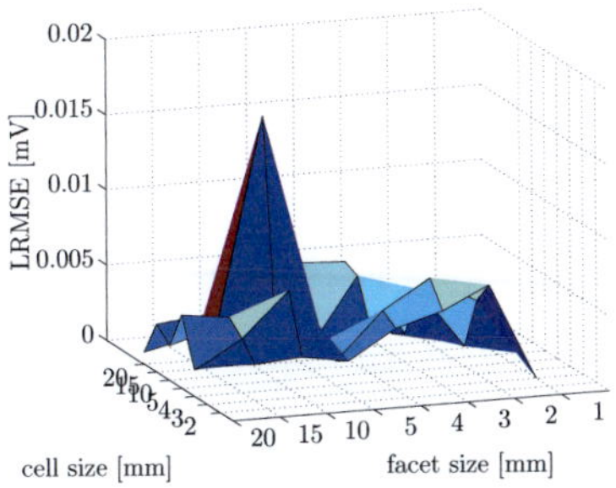

Figure A.8: Realistic thorax model, facet_distance = 0.5 mm. The error in the ECG signal is shown with respect to the case of both the facet and cell size being at their highest resolution in the study. Facet distance is 0.5 mm.

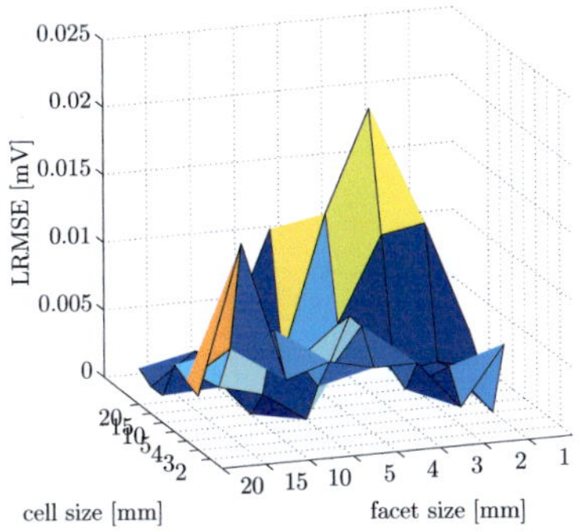

Figure A.9: Realistic thorax model, facet_distance = 1 mm. The error in the ECG signal is shown with respect to the case of both the facet and cell size being at their highest resolution in the study. Facet distance is 1 mm.

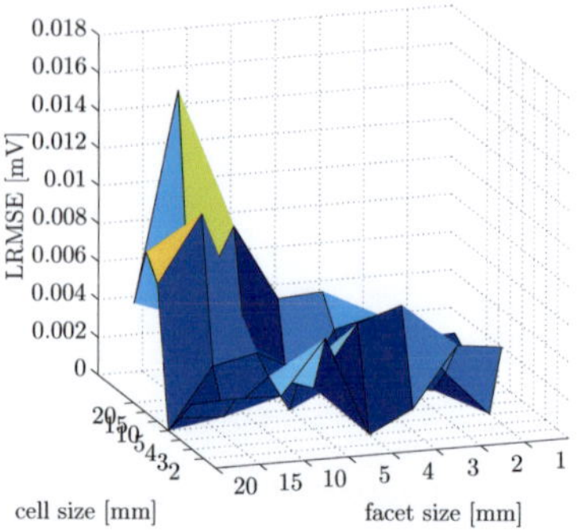

Figure A.10: Realistic thorax model, facet_distance = 5 mm. The error in the ECG signal is shown with respect to the case of both the facet and cell size being at their highest resolution in the study. Facet distance is 5 mm.

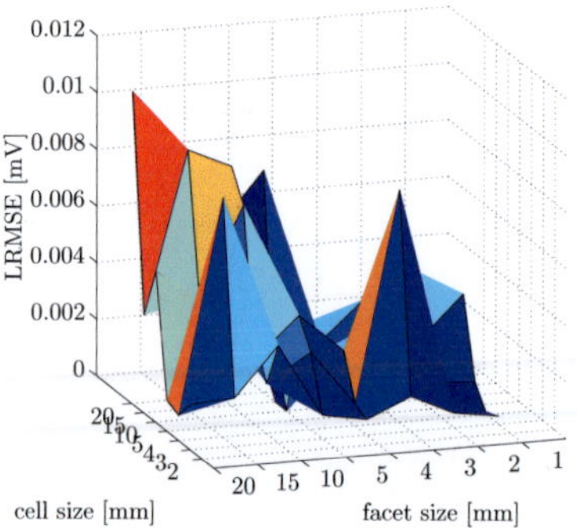

Figure A.11: Realistic thorax model, facet_distance = 10 mm. The error in the ECG signal is shown with respect to the case of both the facet and cell size being at their highest resolution in the study. Facet distance is 10 mm.

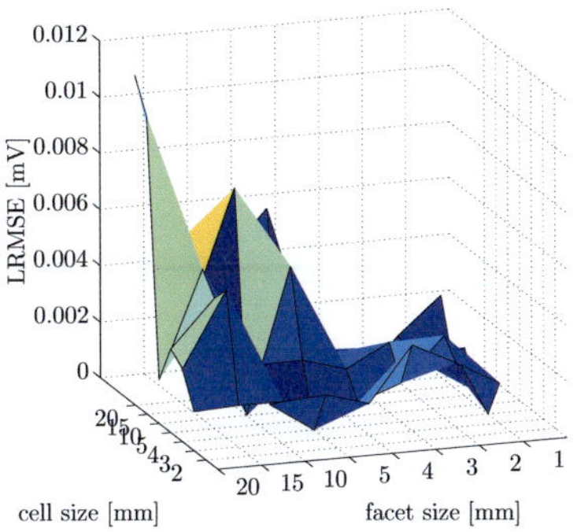

Figure A.12: Realistic thorax model, facet_distance = 16 mm. The error in the ECG signal is shown with respect to the case of both the facet and cell size being at their highest resolution in the study. Facet distance is 16 mm.

A.2.1 Study without Refinement of the Heart

To demonstrate the effects of not working with heart-specific refinement of the mesh, the study with facet_distance of 16 mm was repeated with the meshing parameters for the heart tissue linked to the parameters used in the entire thorax, see Tab. A.4. Results show a much more evident convergence of the produced ECGs with decreasing facet_size and cell_size that is also stronger in amplitude compared to the effects found in the previous studies with realistic thorax model, see Fig. A.13.

Parameter	Range
facet_angle (f_a)	25°
facet_size (f_s)	$[20, 15, 10, 5, 4, \ldots, 1]$ mm
facet_distance (f_d)	16 mm
cell_radius_ edge_ratio (c_r_e)	3
cell_size (c_s)	$[20, 15, 10, 5, 4, 3]$ mm
refine_facet_size (r_f_s)	same as facet_size
refine_cell_size (r_c_s)	same as cell_size

Table A.4: Study without Refinement of the Heart: Variation of Facet Size and Cell Size in Realistic Thorax Model

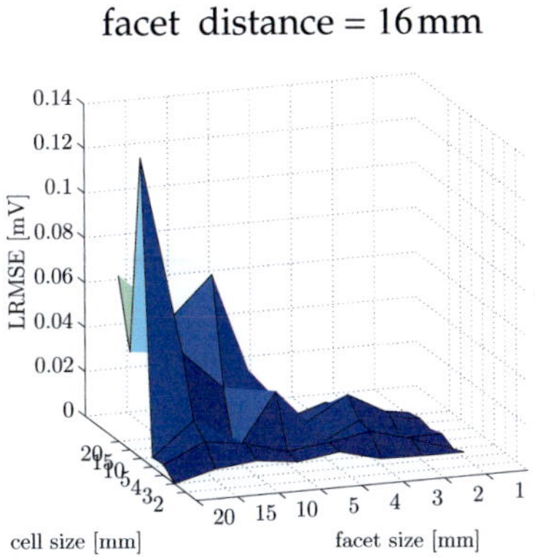

Figure A.13: Realistic thorax model, study without refinement of the heart. The error in the ECG signal is shown with respect to the case of both the facet and cell size being at their highest resolution in the study. Facet distance is 16 mm.

B

Validation Study: Premature Ventricular Contractions

B.1 Description of Datasets

This section features an in-depth description of the datasets presented in Sect. 7.1. Tables provide details on the criteria used for the ratings in Tab. 7.1, see Tab. B.1 for a legend of the quality ratings. Outcomes and durations of ablation therapies are documented in Tab. B.2.

Rating	Description
-	not available/ not performed
x	sufficient quality achieved (partially through manual efforts)
+	OK quality
++	good quality

Table B.1: Legend of quality ratings.

Therapy result	first ablation	last ablation
ablations successful	0h15min	1h54min
	1h16min	2h18min
	0h37min	0h43min
	0h31min	0h47min
ablations, PVC occurrence significantly reduced	0h27min	01h22min
ablations finally not successful	01h31min	03h23min
always paroxysmally treated, then returning, PVC origin sitting too low, presumably	1h15min	2h14min
no ablation performed, risk of an ablation at PVC origin too high	-	(end of the study: 2h44min)
no ablation performed, only a few beats annotated	-	(end of the study: 1h40min)

Table B.2: Outcome and durations of ablation therapies. Each row represents one patient in the study. Patient 08 is not listed, as no invasive study was performed (ablation therapy cancelled).

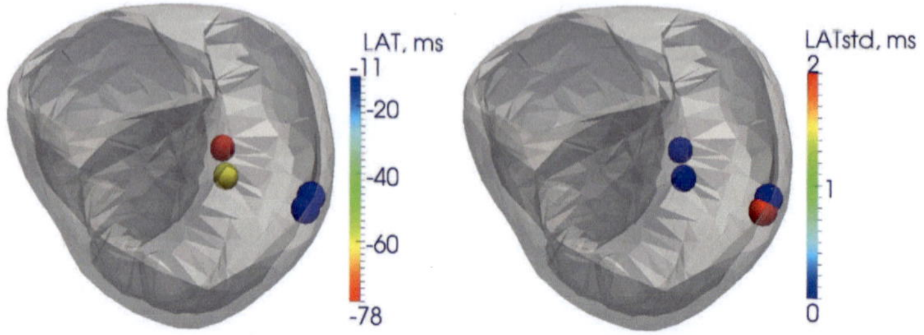

(a) Patient 06, LAT (b) Patient 06, std(LAT)

Figure B.1: Patient 06: Assignment of LAT measurements to the coarse cardiac geometry. Multiple assignments to the same position are averaged (a), with the standard deviation displayed in (b).

Description:	Patient 06, female, PVC diagnosed (LVOT, confirmed in RV mapping). BSPM from MRI session. ablation therapy: without sufficient activity for ablation, not successful

Quality	Step in modeling workflow	Comment
++	Segmentation thorax organs	-
+	Segmentation thorax surface	breast nipples cut off in MRI
++	Segmentation heart	cine MRI
++	Co-registration heart and thorax	heart segmentation fits perfectly well into thorax MRI
+	Electrode localization MackensteinCAM	iPhone 4, corresponding images selected from acquisitions at different times, 8-strip distances: $46.9 \pm 1.3mm$ (45mm), 12-strip distances: $31.2 \pm 0.8mm$ (30mm)
x	Electrode co-registration	Based on very rough position estimates (breast nipples cut off). Registration was corrected manually. 12 back electrodes were integrated in cavities of a mattress and removed during the MRI. The skin relaxed into these cavities during the MRI by approximately 0.5 cm. Positions were corrected accordingly along the anterior-posterior axis.
x	CARTO activation times	6 uncensored measurements (RV) of the PVC (merged into 4 nodes in the coarse mesh representation); no ablations performed.
x	CARTO anatomical map	very little coverage of the RV, landmarks: bundle of His, point in the RVOT
+	CARTO co-registration	distance to endocardial surface: $2.8 \pm 1.5mm$

Table B.3: Patient 06 (ws103-06-P1-F)

Description:	Patien 08, female, sporadic PVC diagnosed (presumably LVOT or RVOT), no CARTO map recorded ablation therapy: cancelled, no therapy performed

Quality	Step in modeling workflow	Comment
++	Segmentation thorax organs	-
+	Segmentation thorax surface	artifact on right shoulder (mostly removed)
++	Segmentation heart	cine MRI
+	Co-registration heart and thorax	RV segmentation extends slightly into the liver, but heart as a whole fits very well into the thorax MRI
+	Electrode localization MackensteinCAM	iPhone 4, corresponding images selected from acquisitions at different times, 8-strip distances: 44.2 ± 3.7 mm (45mm), 12-strip distances: 28.8 ± 2.1 mm (30mm)
x	Electrode co-registration	manual, very difficult (breasts not fully covered by MRI)
-	CARTO activation times	therapy cancelled
-	CARTO anatomical map	therapy cancelled
-	CARTO co-registration	therapy cancelled

Table B.4: Patient 08 (ws103-08-P1-F)

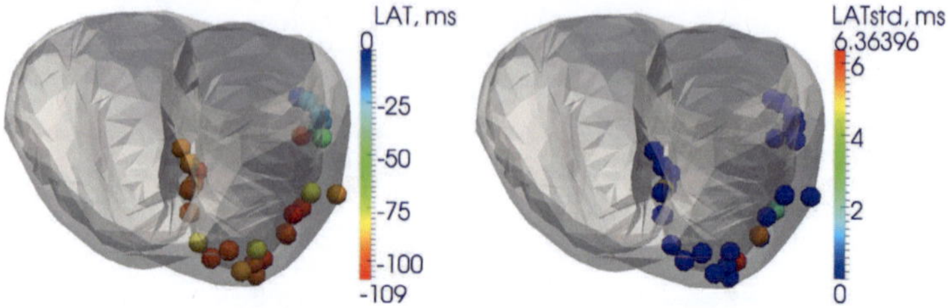

(a) Patient 09, LAT

(b) Patient 09, std(LAT)

Figure B.2: Patient 09: Assignment of LAT measurements to the coarse cardiac geometry. Multiple assignments to the same position are averaged (a), with the standard deviation displayed in (b).

Description:		Patient 09, female, PVC (LV basal/mid-inferoseptal) ablation therapy: successful
Quality	**Step in modeling workflow**	**Comment**
++	Segmentation thorax organs	-
++	Segmentation thorax surface	-
+	Segmentation heart	cine MRI, apex not entirely visible in MRI, step in RV close to base (reasonable, but would profit from confirmation with better image resolution)
+	Co-registration heart and thorax	heart segmentation had to be translated by 30.3 mm to fit well into thorax MRI
+	Electrode localization MackensteinCAM	iPhone 4, corresponding images selected from acquisitions at different times, 8-strip distances: 44.1 ± 2.4 mm (45 mm), 12-strip distances: 29.3 ± 1.8 mm (30 mm).
x	Electrode co-registration	fiducials were of bad accuracy (left breast nipple was close to an artifact, liver spot was only coarsely known and weighted accordingly, a left breast wrinkle, which was also used for co-registration, could only coarsely be localized).
+	CARTO activation times	39 uncensored measurements (LV) of the PVC, but implausibly great area of early activations.
++	CARTO anatomical map	complete coverage of the LV, landmarks: bundle of His, vessel tag of the aorta with corresponding MRI segmentation
+	CARTO co-registration	distance to endocardial surface: $5.0 \pm 3.5 mm$

Table B.5: Patient 09 (ws103-09-P1-F)

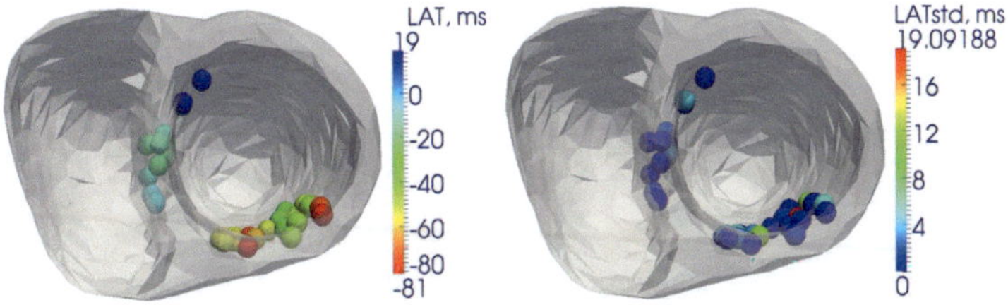

(a) Patient 11, LAT (b) Patient 11, std(LAT)

Figure B.3: Patient 11: Assignment of LAT measurements to the coarse cardiac geometry. Multiple assignments to the same position are averaged (a), with the standard deviation displayed in (b).

	Description:	Patient 11, male, PVC (basal-lateral LV) ablation therapy: presumably not successful (but significantly reduced frequency of PVCs during therapy)
Quality	Step in modeling workflow	Comment
++	Segmentation thorax organs	-
++	Segmentation thorax surface	-
x	Segmentation heart	cine MRI, segmentation with unusual apex, which is in line with the MRI-data and an independent segmentation made by the clinic (potentially due to respiratory effects, as heart motion is not the reason, see cine sequences). RV segmentation closes much lower than the LV at the base (also in line with cine MRI data and segmentation by the clinic).
x	Co-registration heart and thorax	Very bad co-registration. Offset between heart and thorax MRI is not only a translation, but the heart has a different shape (much greater RV chamber in the cine MRI). Correcting the offset by translation: heart segmentation was translated by 14.0mm to fit into thorax MRI.
++	Electrode localization MackensteinCAM	iPhone 4, corresponding images selected from acquisitions at different times, 8-strip distances: 43.8 ± 0.9mm (45mm), 12-strip distances: 29.3 ± 0.8mm (30mm)
x	Electrode co-registration	Electrodes were mapped manually, since apart from the breast nipples, no other landmark could be used.
++	CARTO activation times	65 uncensored measurements (LV) of the PVC
+	CARTO anatomical map	Good coverage of the LV, landmarks: bundle of His, point know to be basal anteriolateral, point know to be basal
++	CARTO co-registration	distance to endocardial surface: 4.5 ± 3.4mm

Table B.6: Patient 11 (ws103-11-P1-M)

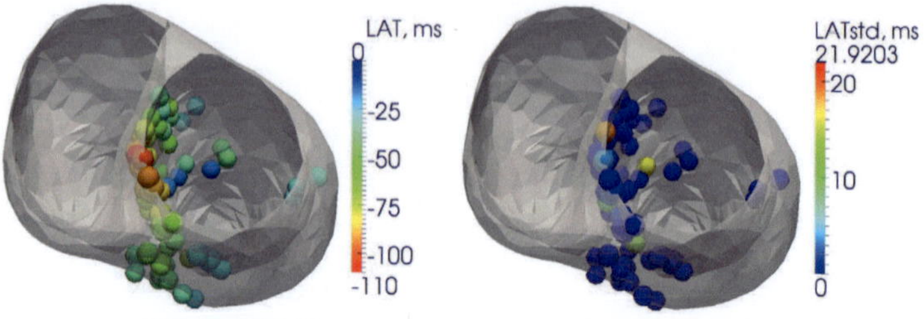

(a) Patient 12, LAT

(b) Patient 12, std(LAT)

Figure B.4: Patient 12: Assignment of LAT measurements to the coarse cardiac geometry. Multiple assignments to the same position are averaged (a), with the standard deviation displayed in (b).

Description:	Patient 12, male, PVC (LVOT, aortomitral) ablation therapy: not successful (no complete suppression of activity)

Quality	Step in modeling workflow	Comment
++	Segmentation thorax organs	-
++	Segmentation thorax surface	-
+	Segmentation heart	cine MRI, good quality only after three cine slices had been ignored in the segmentation
+	Co-registration heart and thorax	heart segmentation was translated by 18.9mm to fit well into thorax MRI
x	Electrode localization MackensteinCAM	iPhone 4, corresponding images selected from acquisitions at different times, 8-strip distances: 37.7 ± 1.9mm (45mm), 12-strip distances: 25.5 ± 0.8mm (30mm). Strong deviation of electrode distances from distance on strips in the real world. However, the distances between the breast nipples marked in the MRI (276.4mm) and in MackensteinCAM (276.6mm) match perfectly well (all coordinates were scaled to a separate metric reference that was placed in the measurement setup).
x	Electrode co-registration	manual, based on breast nipples
++	CARTO activation times	82 uncensored measurements (LV) of the PVC
++	CARTO anatomical map	complete coverage of the LV, landmarks: several bundle of His
+	CARTO co-registration	distance to endocardial surface: 6.8 ± 5.4mm. Many measurements not at the surface, but in the lumen. Very good co-registration from visual impression.

Table B.7: Patient 12 (ws103-12-P1-M)

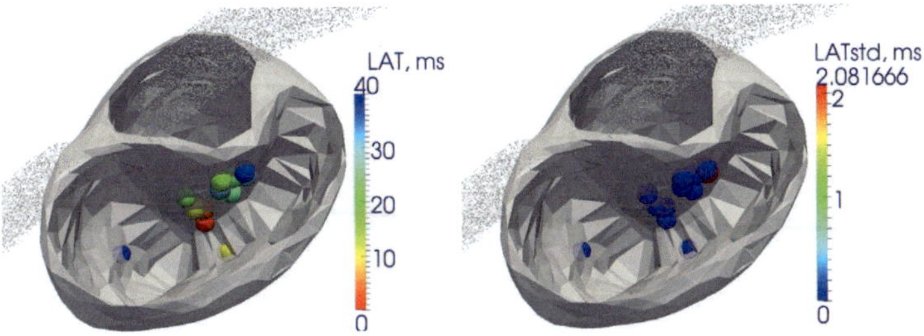

(a) Patient 13, LAT

(b) Patient 13, std(LAT)

Figure B.5: Patient 13: Assignment of LAT measurements (normal sinus rhythm, NSR) to the coarse cardiac geometry. Multiple assignments to the same position are averaged (a), with the standard deviation displayed in (b).

Quality	Step in modeling workflow	Comment
	Description:	Patient 13, female, PVC (RVOT) ablation therapy: successful (significant reduction of activity)
++	Segmentation thorax organs	-
++	Segmentation thorax surface	-
++	Segmentation heart	cine MRI
+	Co-registration heart and thorax	heart segmentation was translated by 11.2 mm to fit well into thorax MRI
++	Electrode localization MackensteinCAM	2 CANON EOS 600D cameras. Left point cloud: 8-strip distances: 44.7 ± 0.2 mm (45 mm), 12-strip distances: 29.8 ± 0.3 mm (30 mm). Right point cloud: 8-strip distances: 44.6 ± 0.3 mm (45 mm), 12-strip distances: 29.9 ± 0.4 mm (30 mm). Scale factor between clouds: 0.99, co-registration error 1.3 ± 0.5 mm
x	Electrode co-registration	registration was corrected manually
+	CARTO activation times	15 uncensored measurements (RV), however, only of normal sinus rhythm (NSR)
+	CARTO anatomical map	locally limited coverage of the RVOT, landmarks: samples from the apex, bundle of His, two vessel tags with corresponding MRI segmentations
++	CARTO co-registration	distance to endocardial surface: 4.0 ± 2.8 mm

Table B.8: Patient 13 (ws103-13-P1-F)

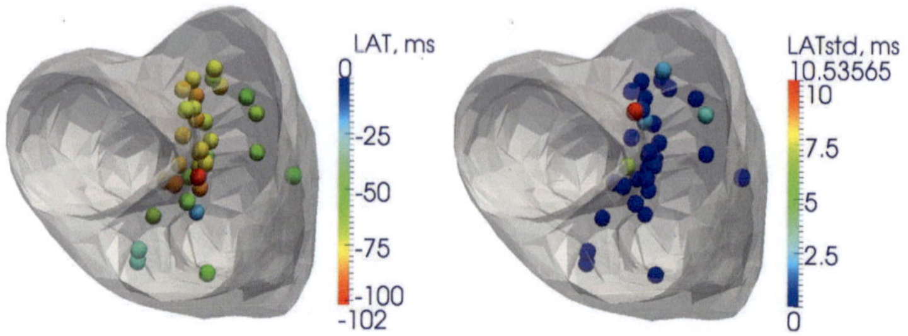

(a) Patient 14, LAT

(b) Patient 14, std(LAT)

Figure B.6: Patient 14: Assignment of LAT measurements to the coarse cardiac geometry. Multiple assignments to the same position are averaged (a), with the standard deviation displayed in (b).

Description:	Patient 14, female, PVC (RV, para-Hisian), follow-up of previous ablation therapy (successful, PVC in LV, under aortic valve, supra-Hisian) ablation therapy: cancelled (origin too close to AV node)

Quality	Step in modeling workflow	Comment
++	Segmentation thorax organs	-
++	Segmentation thorax surface	-
++	Segmentation heart	cine MRI
++	Co-registration heart and thorax	heart segmentation fits well into thorax MRI
++	Electrode localization MackensteinCAM	2 CANON EOS 600D cameras. Left point cloud: 8-strip distances: 43.4 ± 1.0 mm (45 mm), 12-strip distances: 29.0 ± 0.7 mm (30 mm). Right point cloud: 8-strip distances: 44.6 ± 0.3 mm (45 mm) (*), 12-strip distances: 29.4 ± 0.6 mm (30 mm). Scale factor between clouds: 0.99, co-registration error 2.8 ± 1.0 mm.
++	Electrode co-registration	shoulder markers were far off (represented once), but breast nipple markers were reliable (represented 1000 times in the numerical calculations), with very good results
++	CARTO activation times	42 uncensored measurements (RV) of the PVC
++	CARTO anatomical map	complete coverage of the RV, landmarks: two vessel tags with corresponding MRI segmentations, points in the LV
++	CARTO co-registration	distance to endocardial surface: 4.3 ± 3.5 mm

Table B.9: Patient 14 (ws103-14-P1-M)

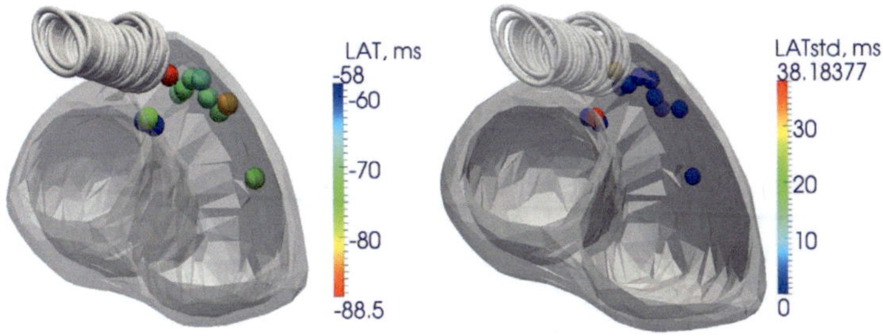

(a) Patient 17, LAT (b) Patient 17, std(LAT)

Figure B.7: Patient 17: Assignment of LAT measurements to the coarse cardiac geometry. Multiple assignments to the same position are averaged (a), with the standard deviation displayed in (b).

Description:	Patient 17, female, PVC (RVOT, septal, below pulmonary valve) ablation therapy: successful

Quality	Step in modeling workflow	Comment
++	Segmentation thorax organs	-
+	Segmentation thorax surface	artifacts ineffective for relevant fields
++	Segmentation heart	cine MRI
+	Co-registration heart and thorax	Heart segmentation was translated by 3.1 mm to fit well into thorax MRI.
++	Electrode localization MackensteinCAM	2 CANON EOS 600D cameras, 8-strip distances: 44.0 ± 1.8 mm (45 mm), 12-strip distances: 29.9 ± 1.1 mm (30 mm).
+	Electrode co-registration	left breast nipple was within an artifact, instead marked by two points that spanned across its assumed position, weighted correct right nipple much stronger than other landmarks, including (with low weighting) the central ends of the clavicles. Resulting fit with thorax surface (cross-check) was very good.
+	CARTO activation times	16 uncensored measurements (RV) of the PVC
+	CARTO anatomical map	RV covered in RVOT area, landmarks: vessel tags
++	CARTO co-registration	distance to endocardial surface: 4.5 ± 2.5 mm

Table B.10: Patient 17 (ws103-17-P1-F)

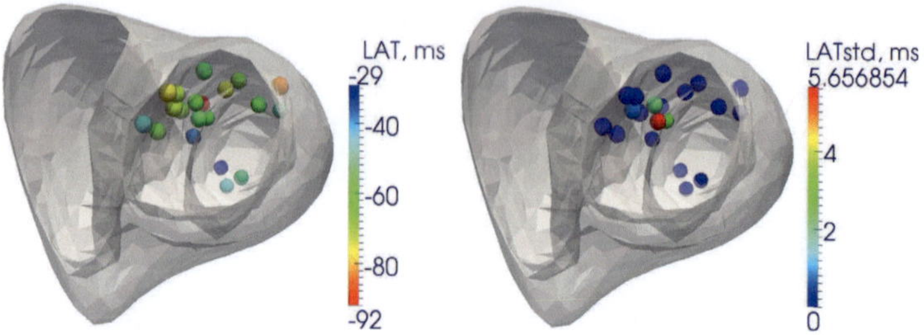

(a) Patient 19, LAT (b) Patient 19, std(LAT)

Figure B.8: Patient 19: Assignment of LAT measurements to the coarse cardiac geometry. Multiple assignments to the same position are averaged (a), with the standard deviation displayed in (b).

Description:	Patient 19, male, PVC (LV, basal infero septal, below mitral valve), follow-up of previous ablation therapy (not successful) ablation therapy: successful

Quality	Step in modeling workflow	Comment
++	Segmentation thorax organs	-
++	Segmentation thorax surface	-
+	Segmentation heart	MR-angiography flash-3d scan (after contrast agent injection) chosen. Mid-septal LV wall unusually thick, but in good correspondence with MRI.
++	Co-registration heart and thorax	heart segmentation fits perfectly well into thorax MRI
++	Electrode localization MackensteinCAM	2 CANON EOS 600D cameras. Left point cloud: 8-strip distances: 44.3 ± 0.0 mm (45 mm), 12-strip distances: 29.8 ± 0.4 mm (30 mm). Right point cloud 8-strip distances: 45.0 ± 0.0 mm (45 mm), 12-strip distances: 29.8 ± 0.7 mm (30 mm). Scale factor between clouds: 0.996, co-registration error 1.4 ± 0.8 mm
+	Electrode co-registration	Corresponding fiducials: L and R breast nipples, liver spot on L breast, tattoo on R arm. Assessment of quality: orthogonal mapping of all 78 positions on the MRI-based thorax surface produced corrections by 7.9 ± 7.6 mm, which was significantly lower for electrodes on the upper (less respiration-affected) part of the body (25% were below 2.1 mm). The maximum distance to the surface was 26.5 mm.
++	CARTO activation times	24 uncensored measurements (LV) of the PVC
++	CARTO anatomical map	complete coverage of the LV, landmarks: two vessel tags with corresponding MRI segmentations
++	CARTO co-registration	distance to endocardial surface: 3.4 ± 2.4 mm

Table B.11: Patient 19 (ws103-19-P1-M)

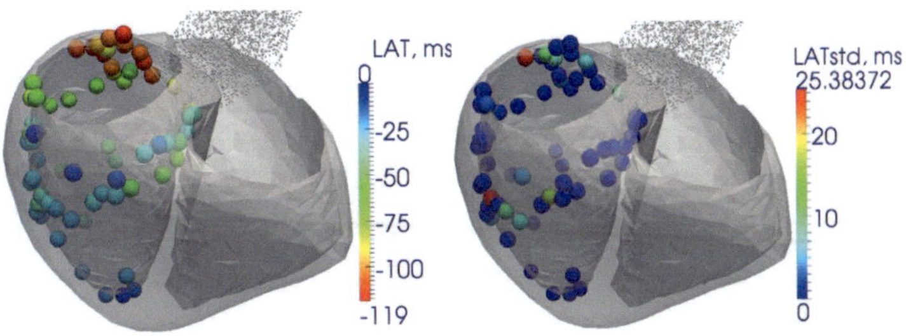

(a) Patient 20, LAT

(b) Patient 20, std(LAT)

Figure B.9: Patient 20: Assignment of LAT measurements to the coarse cardiac geometry. Multiple assignments to the same position are averaged (a), with the standard deviation displayed in (b).

Description:	Patient 20, male, PVC (LVOT, aorta mitral) ablation therapy: successful

Quality	Step in modeling workflow	Comment
++	Segmentation thorax organs	-
++	Segmentation thorax surface	-
++	Segmentation heart	cine MRI
++	Co-registration heart and thorax	heart segmentation fits perfectly well into thorax MRI
++	Electrode localization MackensteinCAM	2 CANON EOS 600D cameras, 8-strip distances: 43.9 ± 0.9 mm (45 mm), 12-strip distances: 28.7 ± 0.5 mm (30 mm).
++	Electrode co-registration	corresponding fiducials: breast nipples (L,R) and 2 liver spots
++	CARTO activation times	88 uncensored measurements (LV) of the PVC
++	CARTO anatomical map	complete coverage of the LV, landmarks: two vessel tags, bundle of HIS
++	CARTO co-registration	distance to endocardial surface: 6.7 ± 4.9 mm, but perfect match by visual judgement

Table B.12: Patient 20 (ws103-20-P1-M)

B.2 ECG Imaging Results

This section includes supplementary ECG imaging results that is referred to from the results chapter (Sect. 7).
Figures B.10, B.11, B.12 and B.13 present localization errors for the Tikhonov method (2nd order, L-curve) for different models (FEM, BEM) and schemes to choose the time of evaluation in the beat (PVC or effective pacing).

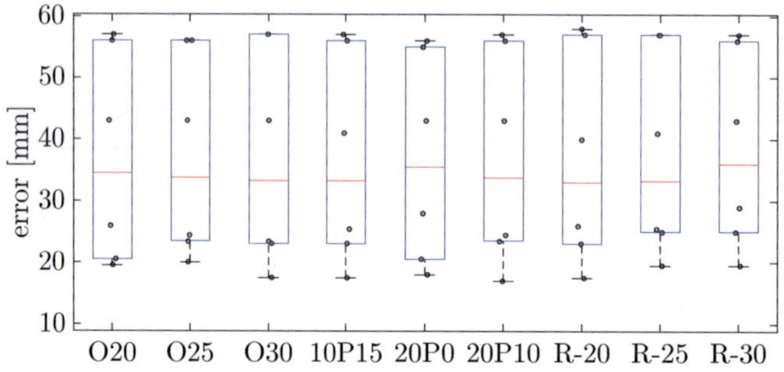

Figure B.10: Localization error (PVCs) for imaged excitation origins (mean 95-percentile [mV] position). Tikhonov method (2nd order, L-curve), FEM-model. Bullets represent median errors for all beats in one of the 10 patients, excluding Patient 06 and Patient 08. Explanation see Sect. 7.1.2 and Fig. 7.5 on page 93.

Fig. B.14 and Fig. B.15 show how results with the Tikhonov (2nd order, FEM-model) depend on the regularization parameter when the R-20 scheme is used to pick the time of evaluation.

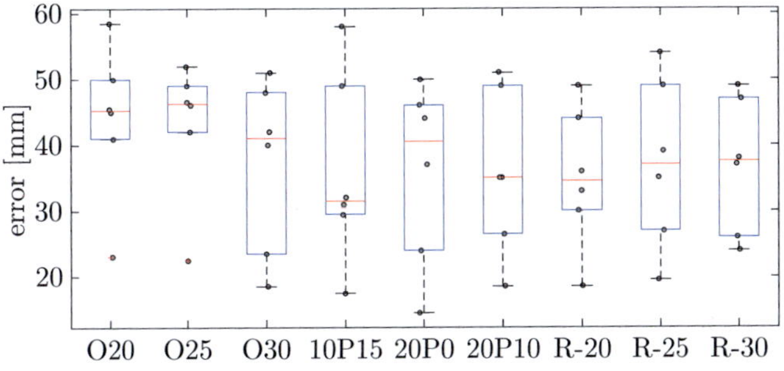

Figure B.11: Localization error (effective pacings) for imaged excitation origins (mean 95-percentile [mV] position). Tikhonov method (2nd order, L-curve), FEM-model. Bullets represent median errors for all beats in one of the 10 patients, excluding Patient 06 and Patient 08. Explanation see Sect. 7.1.2 and Fig. 7.5 on page 93.

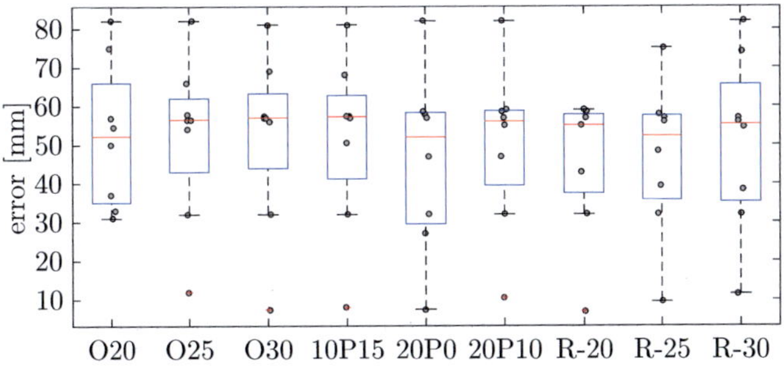

Figure B.12: Localization error (PVCs) for imaged excitation origins (mean 95-percentile [mV] position). Tikhonov method (2nd order, L-curve), BEM-model. Bullets represent median errors for all beats in one of the 10 patients, excluding Patient 06 and Patient 08. Explanation see Sect. 7.1.2 and Fig. 7.5 on page 93.

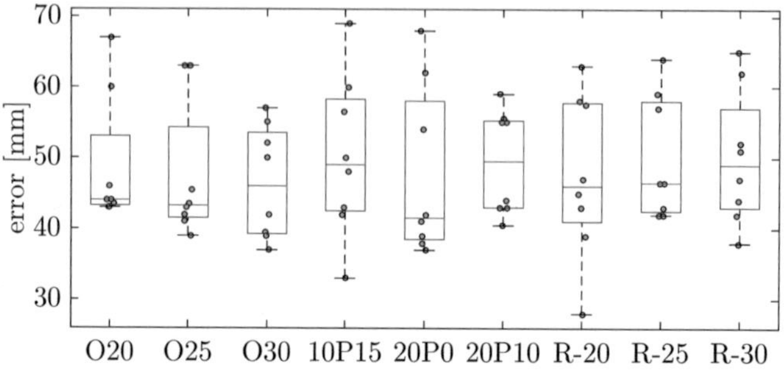

Figure B.13: Localization error (effective pacings) for imaged excitation origins (mean 95-percentile [mV] position). Tikhonov method (2nd order, L-curve), BEM-model. Bullets represent median errors for all beats in one of the 10 patients, excluding Patient 06 and Patient 08. Explanation see Sect. 7.1.2 and Fig. 7.5 on page 93.

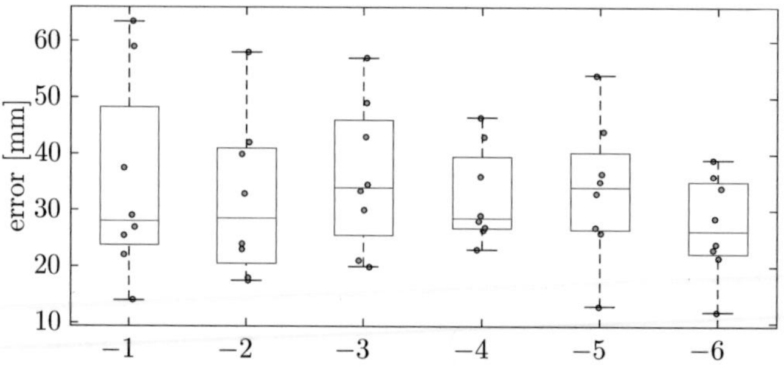

Figure B.14: Tikhonov method (2nd order) over different regularization parameter values (FEM-model, time of evaluation: R-20 scheme). Localization error (PVCs) for imaged excitation origins (mean 95-percentile [mV] position). Bullets represent median errors for all beats in one of the 10 patients, excluding Patient 06 and Patient 08. For further context and information on the results, see Sect. 7.1.2 on page 106.

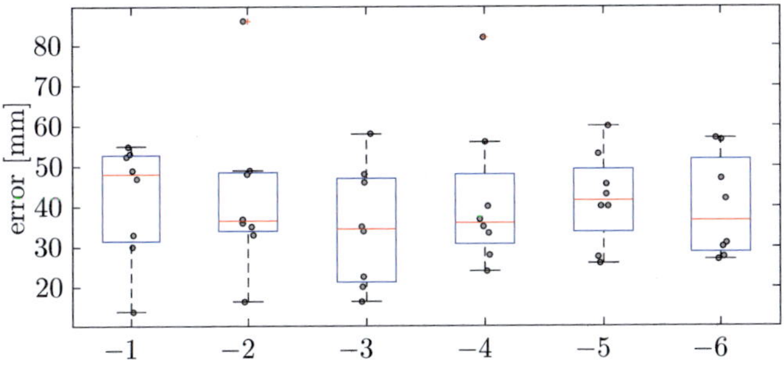

Figure B.15: Tikhonov method (2nd order) over different regularization parameter values (FEM-model, time of evaluation: R-20 scheme). Localization error (effective pacings) for imaged excitation origins (mean 95-percentile [mV] position). Bullets represent median errors for all beats in one of the 10 patients, excluding Patient 06 and Patient 08. For further context and information on the results, see Sect. 7.1.2 on page 106.

References

[1] H. A. Peeters, A. SippensGroenewegen, E. F. Wever, H. Ramanna, A. C. Linnenbank, M. Potse, C. A. Grimbergen, N. M. van Hemel, R. N. Hauer, and E. O. Robles de Medina, "Clinical application of an integrated 3-phase mapping technique for localization of the site of origin of idiopathic ventricular tachycardia," *Circulation*, vol. 99, pp. 1300–1311, 1999.

[2] M. Potse, A. C. Linnenbank, H. A. Peeters, A. SippensGroenewegen, and C. A. Grimbergen, "Continuous localization of cardiac activation sites using a database of multichannel ECG recordings," *IEEE Transactions on Biomedical Engineering*, vol. 47, pp. 682–689, 2000.

[3] R. M. Gulrajani, *Bioelectricity and biomagnetism.* John Wiley & Sons, Inc., 1998.

[4] J. Malmivuo and R. Plonsey, *Bioelectromagnetism. Principles and applications of bioelectric and biomagnetic fields.* New York Oxford: Oxford University Press, 1995.

[5] J. C. Maxwell, "XXV. On physical lines of force," *Philosophical Magazine Series 4*, vol. 21, pp. 161–175, 1861.

[6] W. Lewin, J. Belcher, and P. Dourmashkin, "8.02SC Physics II: Electricity and Magnetism," *Massachusetts Institute of Technology: MIT OpenCourseWare http://ocw.mit.edu (Accessed 03 Feb, 2013). License: Creative Commons BY-NC-SA*, vol. Fall, 2010.

[7] D. J. P. Morris, D. A. Tennant, S. A. Grigera, B. Klemke, C. Castelnovo, R. Moessner, C. Czternasty, M. Meissner, K. C. Rule, J. U. Hoffmann, K. Kiefer, S. Gerischer, D. Slobinsky, and R. S. Perry,

"Dirac Strings and Magnetic Monopoles in the Spin Ice Dy2Ti2O7," *Science*, vol. 326, pp. 411–414, 2009.

[8] O. Tchernyshyov, "Magnetic monopoles: No longer on thin ice," *Nature Physics*, vol. 6, pp. 323–324, 2010.

[9] D. B. Geselowitz, "On the theory of the electrocardiogram," in *Proceddings of the IEEE*, vol. 77, pp. 857–876, IEEE, 1989.

[10] D. B. Geselowitz and T. W. Miller, "A bidomain model for anisotropic cardiac muscle," *Annals of Biomedical Engineering*, vol. 11, pp. 191–206, 1983.

[11] O. Skipa, *Linear inverse problem of electrocardiography: epicardial potentials and transmembrane voltages*. PhD thesis, Helmes Verlag Karlsruhe, 2004.

[12] D. Potyagaylo, M. Segel, W. H. W. Schulze, and O. Dössel, "Non-invasive Localization of Ectopic Foci: a New Optimization Approach for Simultaneous Reconstruction of Transmembrane Voltages and Epicardial Potentials," in *FIMH, LNCS 7945* (S. Ourselin, D. Rueckert, and N. Smith, eds.), pp. 166–173, Spinger-Verlag Berlin Heidelberg, 2013.

[13] D. Potyagaylo, E. G. Cortes, W. H. W. Schulze, and O. Dössel, "Binary optimization for source localization in the inverse problem of ECG," *Medical & Biological Engineering & Computing*, vol. 52, pp. 717–728, 2014.

[14] F. Greensite, "The mathematical basis for imaging cardia electrical function," *Critical Reviews in Biomedical Engineering*, vol. 22, pp. 347–399, 1994.

[15] G. Fischer, B. Tilg, P. Wach, G. Lafer, and W. Rucker, "Analytical validation of the BEM - application of the BEM to the electrocardiographic forward and inverse problem," *Comput Methods Programs Biomed*, vol. 55, pp. 99–106, 1998.

[16] M. Stenroos, V. Mäntynen, and J. Nenonen, "A Matlab library for solving quasi-static volume conduction problems using the boundary element method," *Computer methods and programs in biomedicine*, vol. 88, pp. 256–263, 2007.

[17] U. Kiencke and H. Jäkel, *Signale und Systeme*. München: Oldenbourg-Verl., 2008.

[18] E. Mascarenas Marsal, "Design of Fourier-Based Filters and ECG Templates for Inverse Electrocardiographic Imaging of Patients with Bigeminy," Studienarbeit, Institute of Biomedical Engineering, Karlsruhe Institute of Technology (KIT), 2013.

[19] G. Seemann, D. U. J. Keller, M. W. Krueger, F. M. Weber, M. Wilhelms, and O. Dössel, "Electrophysiological modeling for cardiology: methods and potential applications," *Information Technology*, vol. 52, pp. 242–249, 2010.

[20] M. Stenroos and J. Haueisen, "Boundary element computations in the forward and inverse problems of electrocardiography: comparison of collocation and Galerkin weightings," *Biomedical Engineering, IEEE Transactions on*, vol. 55, pp. 2124–2133, 2008.

[21] D. Farina, *Forward and inverse problems of elctrocardiography: Clinical investigations*. PhD thesis, Karlsruhe, Universitätsverlag Karlsruhe, 2008.

[22] J. S. Hadamard, "Sur les problèmes aux dérivées partielles et leur signification physique," *Princeton University Bulletin*, vol. 13, pp. 49–52, 1902.

[23] W. H. W. Schulze, D. Potyagaylo, and O. Dössel, "Predicting the accuracy of cardiac pace mapping from lead field matrix characteristics," in *Proc. 40th International Congress on Electrocardiology*, 2013.

[24] P. C. Hansen and P. Hansen, eds., *Rank-deficient and discrete ill-posed problems*. Philadelphia: Siam, 1998.

[25] J. J. M. Cuppen and A. Van Oosterom, "Model Studies with the Inversely Calculated lsochrones of Ventricular Depolarization," *IEEE Transactions on Biomedical Engineering*, pp. 652–659, 1984.

[26] W. H. W. Schulze, R. Schimpf, T. Papavassiliu, D. Potyagaylo, E. Tulumen, B. Rudic, V. Liebe, C. Doesch, T. Konrad, C. Veltmann, M. Borggrefe, and O. Dössel, "Electrode arrangements for ECG imaging under practical constraints of a catheter lab setting," in *Biomedizinische Technik / Biomedical Engineering*, vol. 58, 2013.

[27] R. Penrose and J. A. Todd, "On best approximate solutions of linear matrix equations," in *Mathematical Proceedings of the Cambridge Philosophical Society*, vol. 52, pp. 17–19, Cambridge Univ Press, 1956.

[28] P. N. Sabes, "Linear algebraic equations, svd, and the pseudoinverse," 2001.

[29] A. N. Tikhonov and V. Y. Arsenin, *Solutions of ill-posed problem*. Winston&Sons, New York, 1977.

[30] K. B. Petersen and M. S. Pedersen, "The matrix cookbook," *Technical University of Denmark*, 2006.

[31] P. C. Hansen and P. C. O'Leary, "The use of the L-curve in the regularization of discrete ill-posed problems," *SIAM J. Scientific Computing*, vol. 14, pp. 1487–1503, 1993.

[32] P. C. Hansen, "REGULARIZATION TOOLS: A Matlab package for analysis and solution of discrete ill-posed problems," *Numerical Algorithms*, vol. 6, pp. 1–35, 1994.

[33] F. Greensite and G. Huiskamp, "An improved method for estimating epicardial potentials from the body surface," *IEEE Trans. Biomed. Eng.*, vol. 45, pp. 98–104, 1998.

[34] R. Hoekema, "The interindividual variability of the electrocardiogram," Studienarbeit, Katholieke Universiteit Nijmegen, 1999.

[35] R. O. Martin, T. C. Pilkington, and M. N. Morrow, "Statistically constrained inverse electrocardiography," *IEEE Transactions on Biomedical Engineering*, vol. 22, pp. 487–492, 1975.

[36] A. Oosterom van, "The use of the spatial covariance in computing pericardial potentials," *IEEE Trans. Biomed. Eng.*, vol. 46, pp. 778–787, 1999.

[37] Y. Jiang, C. Qian, R. Hanna, D. Farina, and O. Dössel, "Optimization of the electrode positions of multichannel ECG for the reconstruction of ischemic areas by solving the inverse electrocardiographic problem," *International Journal of Bioelectromagnetism (Cover Article)*, vol. 11, pp. 27–37, 2009.

[38] Y. Jiang, *Solving the inverse problem of electrocardiography in a realistic environment*. PhD thesis, KIT Scientific Publishing, 2010.

[39] D. D. Jackson, "The use of a priori data to resolve non-uniqueness in linear inversion," *Geophysical Journal of the Royal Astronomical Society*, vol. 57, pp. 137–157, 1979.

[40] P. M. v. Dam, R. Tung, K. Shivkumar, and M. Laks, "Quantitative localization of premature ventricular contractions using myocardial activation ECGI from the standard 12-lead electrocardiogram," *Journal of Electrocardiology*, vol. 46, pp. 574–579, 2013.

[41] W. H. W. Schulze, D. Potyagaylo, and O. Dössel, "Activation time imaging in the presence of myocardial ischemia: Choice of initial estimates for iterative solvers," in *Computing in Cardiology, 2011*, vol. 39, (9-12 Sept., Krakow), pp. 961–964, 2012.

[42] O. Dössel, Y. Jiang, and W. H. W. Schulze, "Localization of the origin of premature beats using an integral method," in *International Journal of Bioelectromagnetism*, vol. 13, pp. 178–183, 2011.

[43] D. B. Geselowitz, "Use of time integrals of the ECG to solve the inverse problem," *IEEE Trans Biomed Eng*, vol. 32, pp. 73–75, 1985.

[44] R. Modre, B. Tilg, G. Fischer, and P. Wach, "Noninvasive myocardial activation time imaging: a novel inverse algorithm applied to clinical ECG mapping data," *IEEE Trans. Biomed. Eng.*, vol. 49, pp. 1153–1161, 2002.

[45] A. Loewe, W. H. W. Schulze, Y. Jiang, M. Wilhelms, and O. Dössel, "Determination of optimal electrode positions of a wearable ECG monitoring system for detection of myocardial ischemia: a simulation study," in *Computing in Cardiology*, vol. 38, pp. 741–744, 2011.

[46] F. Greensite, "Well-posed formulation of the inverse problem of electrocardiography," *Annals of Biomedical Engineering*, vol. 22, pp. 172–183, 1994.

[47] G. Huiskamp and F. Greensite, "A new method for myocardial activation imaging," *IEEE Trans. Biomed. Eng.*, vol. 44, pp. 433–446, 1997.

[48] M. Seger, B. Pfeifer, and T. Berger, *Electrophysiology - From Plants to Heart*, ch. Noninvasive Imaging of Cardiac Electrophysiology (NICE). InTech, 2012.

[49] A. van Oosterom, "The inverse problem of bioelectricity: an evaluation," *Medical and Biological Engineering and Computing*, vol. 50, pp. 891–902, 2012.

[50] P. W. Macfarlane, A. van Oosterom, O. Pahlm, P. Kligfield, M. Janse, and J. Camm, *Comprehensive electrocardiology*. Springer, 2010.

[51] O. Dössel, "Inverse problem of electro- and magnetocardiography: Review and recent progress," *Int. J. Bioelectromagnetism*, vol. 2, 2000.

[52] R. M. Gulrajani, "The forward and inverse problems of electrocardiography," *IEEE Engineering in Medicine & Biology*, vol. 17, pp. 84–101, 1998.

[53] R. S. MacLeod and D. H. Brooks, "Recent progress in inverse problems in electrocardiology," *IEEE Engineering in Medicine & Biology*, vol. 17, pp. 73–83, 1998.

[54] D. H. Brooks and R. S. MacLeod, "Electrical imaging of the heart," *IEEE Signal Processing Magazine*, vol. 14, pp. 24–42, 1997.

[55] A. Oosterom van, *Computational Biology of the Heart*, ch. Forward and inverse problems in electrocardiography, pp. 295–343. Chichester: John Wiley & Sons, 1997.

[56] C. R. Johnson, "Computational and numerical methods for bioelectric field problems," *Critical Reviews in Biomedical Engineering*, vol. 25, pp. 1–81, 1997.

[57] R. M. Gulrajani, "Models of the electrical activity of the heart and computer simulation of the electrocardiogram," *Crit Rev Biomed Eng*, vol. 16, pp. 1–66, 1988.

[58] Y. Rudy, "Noninvasive electrocardiographic imaging of arrhythmogenic substrates in humans," *Circulation Research*, vol. 112, pp. 863–874, 2013.

[59] C. Ramanathan, R. N. Ghanem, P. Jia, K. Ryu, and Y. Rudy, "Noninvasive electrocardiographic imaging for cardiac electrophysiology and arrhythmia," *Nat Med*, vol. 10, pp. 422–428, 2004.

[60] A. J. Shah, H. S. Lim, S. Yamashita, S. Zellerhoff, B. Berte, S. Mahida, D. Hooks, N. Aljefairi, N. Derval, A. Denis, F. Sacher,

P. Jais, R. Dubois, M. Hocini, and M. Haissaguerre, "Non-Invasive ECG Mapping To Guide Catheter Ablation," *Journal of Atrial Fibrillation*, vol. 7, pp. 31–38, 2014.

[61] A. S. Revishvili, V. V. Kalinin, and A. V. Kalinin, "Method of noninvasive electrophysiological study of the heart," 2013.

[62] R. Tilz, C. Lemes, T. Lin, E. Wissner, A. Rillig, A. Metzner, S. Mathew, F. Ouyang, and K. Kuck, *Europace*, vol. 16, ch. Comparison of Atrial Fibrillation Rotors Identified by Endocardial versus Epicardial Rotor Mapping. 2014.

[63] L. A. Bokeriya, A. S. Revishvili, A. V. Kalinin, V. V. Kalinin, O. A. Lyadzhina, and E. A. Fetisova, "Hardware?Software System for Noninvasive Electrocardiographic Heart Examination Based on Inverse Problem of Electrocardiography," *Biomedical engineering*, vol. 42, pp. 273–279, 2008.

[64] A. M. Denisov, E. V. Zakharov, A. V. Kalinin, and V. V. Kalinin, "Numerical solution of an inverse electrocardiography problem for a medium with piecewise constant electrical conductivity," *Computational Mathematics and Mathematical Physics*, vol. 50, pp. 1172–1177, 2010.

[65] B. Erem, J. Coll-Font, R. Martinez Orellana, P. Stovicek, and D. H. Brooks, "Using Transmural Regularization and Dynamic Modeling for Non-Invasive Cardiac Potential Imaging of Endocardial Pacing with Imprecise Thoracic Geometry," *Medical Imaging, IEEE Transactions on*, vol. 33, pp. 726–738, 2014.

[66] Y. Wang, P. S. Cuculich, J. Zhang, K. A. Desouza, R. Vijayakumar, J. Chen, M. N. Faddis, B. D. Lindsay, T. W. Smith, and Y. Rudy, "Noninvasive electroanatomic mapping of human ventricular arrhythmias with electrocardiographic imaging," *Science Translational Medicine*, vol. 3, p. 98ra84, 2011.

[67] R. N. Ghanem, P. Jia, C. Ramanathan, K. Ryu, A. Markowitz, and Y. Rudy, "Noninvasive electrocardiographic imaging (ECGI): comparison to intraoperative mapping in patients," *Heart Rhythm*, vol. 2, pp. 339–354, 2005.

[68] B. Tilg, G. Fischer, R. Modre, F. Hanser, B. Messnarz, M. Schocke, C. Kremser, T. Berger, F. Hintringer, and F. X. Roithinger, "Model-based imaging of cardiac electrical excitation in humans," *IEEE Transactions on Medical Imaging*, vol. 21, pp. 1031–1039, 2002.

[69] T. Berger, B. Pfeifer, F. F. Hanser, F. Hintringer, G. Fischer, M. Netzer, T. Trieb, M. Stuehlinger, W. Dichtl, C. Baumgartner, O. Pachinger, and M. Seger, "Single-beat noninvasive imaging of ventricular endocardial and epicardial activation in patients undergoing CRT," *PloS one*, vol. 6, p. e16255, 2011.

[70] S. Yuan, P. Blomstrom, S. Pehrson, and S. B. Olsson, "Localization of cardiac arrhythmias: conventional noninvasive methods," *International Journal of Cardiac Imaging*, vol. 7, pp. 193–205, 1991.

[71] M. P. Nash and A. J. Pullan, "Challenges Facing Validation of Noninvasive Electrical Imaging of the Heart," *Annals of Noninvasive Electrocardiology*, vol. 10, pp. 73–82, 2005.

[72] A. Intini, R. N. Goldstein, P. Jia, C. Ramanathan, K. Ryu, B. Giannattasio, R. Gilkeson, B. S. Stambler, P. Brugada, W. G. Stevenson, Y. Rudy, and A. L. Waldo, "Electrocardiographic imaging (ECGI), a novel diagnostic modality used for mapping of focal left ventricular tachycardia in a young athlete," *Heart Rhythm : the Official Journal of the Heart Rhythm Society*, vol. 2, pp. 1250–1252, 2005.

[73] J. L. Sapp, F. Dawoud, J. C. Clements, and B. M. Horácek, "Inverse Solution Mapping of Epicardial Potentials Quantitative Comparison With Epicardial Contact Mapping," *Circulation: Arrhythmia and Electrophysiology*, vol. 5, pp. 1001–1009, 2012.

[74] T. Berger, G. Fischer, B. Pfeifer, R. Modre, F. Hanser, T. Trieb, F. X. Roithinger, M. Stuehlinger, O. Pachinger, B. Tilg, and F. Hintringer, "Single-beat noninvasive imaging of cardiac electrophysiology of ventricular pre-excitation," *J. Am. Coll. Cardiol.*, vol. 48, pp. 2045–2052, 2006.

[75] F. Hanser, B. Tilg, R. Modre, G. Fischer, B. Messnarz, F. Hintringer, and F. X. Roithinger, "Feasibility of atrial activation time imaging," in *Proc. Computers in Cardiology*, vol. 29, pp. 601–604, IEEE, 2002.

[76] R. Modre, B. Tilg, G. Fischer, F. Hanser, B. Messnarz, M. Seger, M. F. H. Schocke, T. Berger, F. Hintringer, and F. X. Roithinger, "Atrial noninvasive activation mapping of paced rhythm data," *Journal of Cardiovascular Electrophysiology*, vol. 14, pp. 712–719, 2003.

[77] D. Lai, J. Sun, Y. Li, and B. He, "Usefulness of ventricular endocardial electric reconstruction from body surface potential maps to noninvasively localize ventricular ectopic activity in patients," *Physics in Medicine and Biology*, vol. 58, pp. 3897–3909, 2013.

[78] R. S. MacLeod, M. Gardner, R. M. Miller, and B. M. Horacek, "Application of an electrocardiographic inverse solution to localize ischemia during coronary angioplasty," *J Cardiovasc Electrophysiol*, vol. 6, pp. 2–18, 1995.

[79] P. M. van Dam, T. F. Oostendorp, A. C. Linnenbank, and A. van Oosterom, "Non-invasive imaging of cardiac activation and recovery," *Annals of Biomedical Engineering*, vol. 37, pp. 1739–1756, 2009.

[80] D. Farina, Y. Jiang, O. Dössel, C. Kaltwasser, and W. R. Bauer, "Model-based method of non-invasive reconstruction of ectopic focus locations in the left ventricle," in *Proc. the 4th European Congress for Medical and Biomedical Engineering* (P. V. J. Vander Sloten, ed.), pp. 2560–2563, Springer-Verlag Berlin Heidelberg, 2008.

[81] D. Farina and O. Dössel, "Non-invasive model-based localization of ventricular ectopic centers from multichannel ECG," *International Journal of Applied Electromagnetics and Mechanics*, vol. 30, pp. 289–297, 2009.

[82] Z. Liu, C. Liu, and B. He, "Noninvasive reconstruction of three-dimensional ventricular activation sequence from the inverse solution of distributed equivalent current density," *IEEE Trans Med Imaging*, vol. 25, pp. 1307–1318, 2006.

[83] S. Ohyu, Y. Okamoto, and S. Kuriki, "Use of the ventricular propagated excitation model in the magnetocardiographic inverse problem for reconstruction of electrophysiological properties," *IEEE Transactions on Biomedical Engineering*, vol. 49, pp. 509–519, 2002.

[84] W. Schulze, "Noninvasive reconstruction of cardiac electrophysiology using the Kalman filter," Diplomarbeit, Institut für Biomedizinische Technik, Karlsruher Institut für Technologie (KIT), Karlsruhe, 2009.

[85] W. H. W. Schulze, D. U. J. Keller, and O. Dössel, "A recursive cellular automaton that reconstructs transmembrane voltages with a range-adjusted Tikhonov-method," in *International Journal of Bioelectromagnetism*, vol. 13, pp. 184–189, 2011.

[86] W. H. W. Schulze, F. Elies Henar, D. Potyagaylo, A. Loewe, M. Stenroos, and O. Dössel, "Kalman Filter with Augmented Measurement Model: an ECG Imaging Simulation Study," in *FIMH, LNCS 7945* (S. Ourselin, D. Rueckert, and N. Smith, eds.), pp. 200–207, Springer-Verlag Berlin Heidelberg, 2013.

[87] L. Wang, H. Zhang, K. Wong, H. Liu, and P. Shi, "Physiological-Model-Constrained Noninvasive Reconstruction of Volumetric Myocardial Transmembrane Potentials," *Biomedical Engineering, IEEE Transactions on*, vol. 57, pp. 296–315, 2010.

[88] R. R. Aliev and A. V. Panfilov, "A simple two-variable model of cardiac excitation," *Chaos, Solitons & Fractals*, vol. 7, pp. 293–301, 1996.

[89] D. Potyagaylo, W. H. W. Schulze, and O. Dössel, "Solving the transmembrane potential based inverse problem of ECG under physiological constraints on the solution range," in *Biomedizinische Technik / Biomedical Engineering*, vol. 57, p. 170, 2012.

[90] W. H. W. Schulze, B. Wang, D. Potyagaylo, and O. Dössel, "Use of a tolerance operator in wavefront-based ECG imaging of transmembrane voltages," in *IFMBE Proceedings World Congress on Medical Physics and Biomedical Engineering*, vol. 39, 2012.

[91] W. H. W. Schulze, M. W. Krueger, K. Rhode, R. Razavi, and O. Dössel, "Critical times based activation time imaging," in *Proc. 38th International Congress on Electrocardiology*, 2011.

[92] M. C. Grant and S. P. Boyd, *Recent advances in learning and control*, ch. Graph implementations for nonsmooth convex programs, pp. 95–110. Springer, 2008.

[93] I. CVX Research, "CVX: Matlab Software for Disciplined Convex Programming, version 2.0 beta," 2012.

[94] T. Jokiniemi, K. Simelius, J. Nenonen, I. Tierala, L. Toivonen, and T. Katilal, "Baseline reconstruction for localization of rapid ventricular tachycardia from body surface potential maps," *Physiological Measurement*, vol. 24, pp. 641–651, 2003.

[95] T. Jokiniemi, K. Simelius, J. Nenonen, L. Toivonen, and T. Katila, "An electrocardiographic baseline reconstruction method for rapid ventricular tachycardia," in *Computers in Cardiology 1997*, pp. 251–254, 1997.

[96] F. Greensite, "The temporal prior in bioelectromagnetic source imaging problems," *Biomedical Engineering, IEEE Transactions on*, vol. 50, pp. 1152–1159, 2003.

[97] S. A. Niederer, E. Kerfoot, A. P. Benson, M. O. Bernabeu, O. Bernus, C. Bradley, E. M. Cherry, R. Clayton, F. H. Fenton, A. Garny, E. Heidenreich, S. Land, M. Maleckar, P. Pathmanathan, G. Plank, J. F. Rodriguez, I. Roy, F. B. Sachse, G. Seemann, O. Skavhaug, and N. P. Smith, "Verification of cardiac tissue electrophysiology simulators using an N-version benchmark," *Philosophical Transactions of the Royal Society A: Mathematical, Physical and Engineering Sciences*, vol. 369, pp. 4331–4351, 2011.

[98] M. Karl, G. Seemann, F. Sachse, O. Dössel, and V. Heuveline, "Time and memory efficient implementation of the cardiac bidomain equations," in *4th European Conference of the International Federation for Medical and Biological Engineering, IFMBE Proceedings*, vol. 22, Springer Berlin heidelberg, 2008.

[99] G. Shou, L. Xia, M. Jiang, Q. Wei, F. Liu, and S. Crozier, "Truncated Total Least Squares: A New Regularization Method for the Solution of ECG Inverse Problems," *Biomedical Engineering, IEEE Transactions on*, vol. 55, pp. 1327–1335, 2008.

[100] A. C. Metting van Rijn, A. Peper, and C. A. Grimbergen, "High-quality recording of bioelectric events. Part 2. Low-noise, low-power multichannel amplifier design," *Medical & Biological Engineering & Computing*, vol. 29, pp. 433–440, 1991.

[101] A. C. MettingVanRijn, A. P. Kuiper, T. E. Dankers, and C. A. Grimbergen, "Low-cost active electrode improves the resolution in biopotential recordings," in *Engineering in Medicine and Biology Society, 1996. Bridging Disciplines for Biomedicine. Proceedings of the 18th Annual International Conference of the IEEE*, vol. 1, pp. 101–102, 1996.

[102] Y. Jiang, D. Farina, and O. Dössel, "Reconstruction of myocardial infarction using the improved spatio-temporal MAP-based regularization," in *Proc. the 6th International Symposium on Noninvasive Functional Source Imaging of the Brain and Heart and the International Conference on Functional Biomedical Imaging*, 2007.

[103] R. Miri, I. M. Graf, J. V. Bayarri, and O. Dössel, "Applicability of body surface potential map in computerized optimization of biventricular pacing," *Annals of Biomedical Engineering*, vol. 38, pp. 865–875, 2010.

[104] D. Keller, *Multiscale modeling of the ventricles: From cellular electrophysiology to body surface electrocardiograms*. PhD thesis, Karlsruhe, KIT Scientific Publishing, 2011.

[105] M. W. Krueger, G. Seemann, K. Rhode, D. U. J. Keller, C. Schilling, A. Arujuna, J. Gill, M. D. O'Neill, R. Razavi, and O. Dossel, "Personalization of atrial anatomy and electrophysiology as a basis for clinical modeling of radio-frequency ablation of atrial fibrillation," *IEEE Transactions on Medical Imaging*, vol. 32, pp. 73–84, 2013.

[106] I. B. A. Menown, "Body surface mapping: potential role in a chest pain critical care pathway," *Critical Pathways in Cardiology*, vol. 2, pp. 46–51, 2003.

[107] C. G. Owens, A. J. J. McClelland, S. J. Walsh, B. A. Smith, A. Tomlin, J. W. Riddell, M. Stevenson, and A. A. J. Adgey, "Prehospital 80-LAD mapping: does it add significantly to the diagnosis of acute coronary syndromes?," *Journal of Electrocardiology*, vol. 37 Suppl, pp. 223–232, 2004.

[108] J. Blechert, J. E. Goltsche, B. M. Herbert, and F. H. Wilhelm, "Eat your troubles away: electrocortical and experiential correlates of food image processing are related to emotional eating style and

emotional state," *Biological Psychology*, vol. 96, pp. 94–101, 2014.

[109] C. v. d. Steeg, A. Daffertshofer, D. F. Stegeman, and T. W. Boonstra, "High-density surface electromyography improves the identification of oscillatory synaptic inputs to motoneurons," *Journal of Applied Physiology (Bethesda, Md. : 1985)*, vol. 116, pp. 1263–1271, 2014.

[110] M. YingLiang, U. Mistry, A. Thorpe, R. J. Housden, Z. Chen, W. H. W. Schulze, C. A. Rinaldi, R. Razavi, and K. Rhode, "Automatic Electrode and CT/MR Image Co-localisation for Electrocardiographic Imaging," in *FIMH, LNCS 7945* (S. Ourselin, D. Rueckert, and N. Smith, eds.), pp. 268–275, Springer-Verlag berlin Heidelberg, 2013.

[111] A. Thorpe, Z. Chen, W. H. W. Schulze, M. W. Krueger, J. Relan, H. Delin-gette, R. Razavi, C. Rinaldi, and K. Rhode, "Enhanced workflow for BSPM and ECGi using X-ray based Electrode Localisation," in *Bioengineering12*, 2012.

[112] W. H. W. Schulze, P. Mackens, D. Potyagaylo, K. Rhode, E. Tulumen, R. Schimpf, T. Papavassiliu, M. Borggrefe, and O. Dössel, "Automatic camera-based identification and 3-D reconstruction of electrode positions in electrocardiographic imaging," *Biomedizinische Technik. Biomedical Engineering*, 2014.

[113] J. E. Burnes, B. Taccardi, R. S. MacLeod, and Y. Rudy, "Noninvasive ECG imaging of electrophysiologically abnormal substrates in infarcted hearts : A model study," *Circulation*, vol. 101, pp. 533–540, 2000.

[114] J. E. Burnes, B. Taccardi, and Y. Rudy, "A noninvasive imaging modality for cardiac arrhythmias," *Circulation*, vol. 102, pp. 2152–2158, 2000.

[115] R. N. Ghanem, J. E. Burnes, A. L. Waldo, and Y. Rudy, "Imaging dispersion of myocardial repolarization, II: noninvasive reconstruction of epicardial measures," *Circulation*, vol. 104, pp. 1306–1312, 2001.

[116] L. Cheng, *Non-invasive electrical imaging of the heart*. PhD thesis, University of Auckland, 2001.

[117] P. Mackens and W. H. W. Schulze, "MackensteinCAM (https://github.com/IBTKIT/MackensteinCAM)," 2014.

[118] K. S. Rhode, D. L. G. Hill, P. J. Edwards, J. Hipwell, D. Rueckert, G. Sanchez-Ortiz, S. Hegde, V. Rahunathan, and R. Razavi, "Registration and tracking to integrate X-ray and MR images in an XMR facility," *IEEE Transactions on Medical Imaging*, vol. 22, pp. 1369–1378, 2003.

[119] M. W. Krueger, *Personalized Multi-Scale Modeling of the Atria: Heterogeneities, Fiber Architecture, Hemodialysis and Ablation Therapy*. PhD thesis, Karlsruhe, KIT Scientific Publishing, 2012.

[120] R. I. Hartley and A. Zisserman, *Multiple View Geometry in Computer Vision*. Cambridge, United Kingdom: Cambridge University Press, 2004.

[121] R. N. Ghanem, C. Ramanathan, P. Jia, and Y. Rudy, "Heart-surface reconstruction and ECG electrodes localization using fluoroscopy, epipolar geometry and stereovision: application to noninvasive imaging of cardiac electrical activity," *IEEE Transactions on Medical Imaging*, vol. 22, pp. 1307–1318, 2003.

[122] J. J. M. Cuppen, "Calculating the isochrones of ventricular depolarization," *SIAM Journal on Scientific and Statistical Computing*, vol. 5, p. 105, 1984.

[123] A. D. Scott, J. Keegan, and D. N. Firmin, "Motion in cardiovascular MR imaging," *Radiology*, vol. 250, pp. 331–351, 2009.

[124] H. J. Michealy and S. O. Schoenberg, "MAGNETOM Skyra: The Mannheim Perspective, journal=MAGNETOM flash," pp. 24–30, 2011.

[125] R. L. Ehman and J. P. Felmlee, "Adaptive technique for high-definition MR imaging of moving structures," *Radiology*, vol. 173, pp. 255–263, 1989.

[126] M. Szimtenings and Siemens Medical Solutions, "Motion under Control with Prospective Acquisition Correction (PACE)," tech. rep., 2012.

[127] P. Zerfass, F. B. Sachse, C. D. Werner, and O. Dössel, "Deformation of surface nets for interactive segmentation of tomographic data,"

in *Biomedizinische Technik*, vol. 45-1, pp. 483–484, 2000.

[128] A. Fedorov, R. Beichel, J. Kalpathy-Cramer, J. Finet, J.-C. Fillion-Robin, S. Pujol, C. Bauer, D. Jennings, F. Fennessy, M. Sonka, J. Buatti, S. Aylward, J. V. Miller, S. Pieper, and R. Kikinis, "3D Slicer as an image computing platform for the Quantitative Imaging Network," *Magnetic Resonance Imaging*, vol. 30, pp. 1323–1341, 2012.

[129] S. Pieper, M. Halle, and R. Kikinis, "3D Slicer," in *Biomedical Imaging: Nano to Macro, 2004. IEEE International Symposium on*, vol. Vol. 1, pp. 632–635, IEEE, 2004.

[130] R. Prakash, "Determination of right ventricular wall thickness in systole and diastole. Echocardiographic and necropsy correlation in 32 patients," *British Heart Journal*, vol. 40, pp. 1257–1261, 1978.

[131] L. G. Rudski, W. W. Lai, J. Afilalo, L. Hua, M. D. Handschumacher, K. Chandrasekaran, S. D. Solomon, E. K. Louie, and N. B. Schiller, "Guidelines for the echocardiographic assessment of the right heart in adults: a report from the American Society of Echocardiography endorsed by the European Association of Echocardiography, a registered branch of the European Society of Cardiology, and the Canadian Society of Echocardiography," *Journal of the American Society of Echocardiography : Official Publication of the American Society of Echocardiography*, vol. 23, pp. 685–713; quiz 786, 2010.

[132] S. Y. Ho and P. Nihoyannopoulos, "Anatomy, echocardiography, and normal right ventricular dimensions," *Heart (British Cardiac Society)*, vol. 92 Suppl 1, pp. i2–13, 2006.

[133] S. Y. Ho, "Anatomy and myoarchitecture of the left ventricular wall in normal and in disease," *European Journal of Echocardiography : the Journal of the Working Group on Echocardiography of the European Society of Cardiology*, vol. 10, pp. iii3–7, 2009.

[134] F. B. Sachse, M. Glas, M. Müller, and K. Meyer-Waarden, "Segmentation and Tissue-Classification of the Visible Man Dataset Using the Computertomographic Scans and the Thin-Section Photos," in *Proc. First Users Conference of the National Library of Medicines*

Visible Human Project, 1996.

[135] C. Werner, F. Sachse, and O. Dössel, "Applications of the visible human male dataset in electrocardiology: simulation of the electrical excitation propagation," in *Proceedings of 2nd User Conference of the National Liberary of Medicines Visible Human Project*, pp. 69–70, 1998.

[136] O. Ecabert, J. Peters, H. Schramm, C. Lorenz, J. von Berg, M. J. Walker, M. Vembar, M. E. Olszewski, K. Subramanyan, G. Lavi, and J. Weese, "Automatic model-based segmentation of the heart in CT images," *IEEE Transactions on Medical Imaging*, vol. 27, pp. 1189–1201, 2008.

[137] Z. Chen, J. Relan, W. Schulze, R. Karim, M. Sohal, A. Shetty, Y. L. Ma, N. Ayache, M. Sermesant, H. Delingette, J. Bostock, R. Razavi, K. Rhode, and A. Rinaldi, "Simultaneous non-contact mapping fused with CMR derived grey zone to explore the relationship with ventricular tachycardia substrate in ischaemic cardiomyopathy," in *Journal of Cardiovascular Magnetic Resonance*, vol. 15, p. P64, 2013.

[138] B. He, G. Li, and X. Zhang, "Noninvasive three-dimensional activation time imaging of ventricular excitation by means of a heart-excitation model," *Physics in medicine and biology*, vol. 47, pp. 4063–4078, 2002.

[139] "Computational geometry algorithms library (www.cgal.org)."

[140] D. D. Streeter, *Handbook of Physiology. Section 2: The Cardiovascular System*, vol. Vol. I. The Heart, ch. Gross morphology and fiber geometry of the heart, pp. 61–112. Baltimore: Williams and Wilkins: American Physiology Socienty, 1979.

[141] S. Gabriel, R. W. Lau, and C. Gabriel, "The dielectric properties of biological tissues: II. Measurements in the frequency range 10 Hz to 20 GHz," *Physics in Medicine and Biology*, vol. 41, pp. 2251–2269, 1996.

[142] W. H. W. Schulze, T. Fritz, D. Potyagaylo, J. Trächtler, R. Schimpf, T. Papavassiliu, E. Tülümen, B. Rudic, V. Liebe, C. Doesch, M. Borggrefe, and O. Dössel, "Effect of mesh resolution on for-

ward calculations of the electrocardiogram in a simplified thorax model," in *Biomedizinische Technik / Biomedical Engineering*, vol. 59, pp. 945–948, 2014.

[143] D. Swenson, J. Levine, Z. Fu, J. Tate, and R. MacLeod, "The effect of non-conformal finite element boundaries on electrical monodomain and bidomain simulations," in *Computing in Cardiology, 2010*, pp. 97–100, 2010.

[144] P. Cignoni, M. Corsini, and G. Ranzuglia, "Meshlab: an open-source 3d mesh processing system," *Ercim news*, vol. 73, pp. 45–46, 2008.

[145] P. J. Besl and H. D. Mckay, "A method for registration of 3-D shapes," *Pattern Analysis and Machine Intelligence, IEEE Transactions on*, vol. 14, pp. 239–256, 1992.

[146] K. S. Arun, T. S. Huang, and S. D. Blostein, "Least-squares fitting of two 3-D point sets," *IEEE Transactions on Pattern Analysis and Machine Intelligence*, vol. 9, pp. 698–700, 1987.

[147] K. Vetters, *Formeln und Fakten im Grundkurs Mathematik*. 2004.

[148] A. C. Metting van Rijn, A. Peper, and C. A. Grimbergen, "High-quality recording of bioelectric events. Part 1. Interference reduction, theory and practice," *Medical & Biological Engineering & Computing*, vol. 28, pp. 389–397, 1990.

[149] G. Fischer, B. Tilg, R. Modre, F. Hanser, B. Messnarz, and P. Wach, "On modeling the wilson terminal in the boundary and finite element method," *IEEE Transactions on Biomedical Engineering*, vol. 49, pp. 217–224, 2002.

[150] G. Fischer, F. Hanser, B. Pfeifer, M. Seger, C. Hintermuller, R. Modre, B. Tilg, T. Trieb, T. Berger, F. X. Roithinger, and F. Hintringer, "A signal processing pipeline for noninvasive imaging of ventricular preexcitation," *Methods of Information in Medicine*, vol. 44, pp. 508–515, 2005.

[151] K. Rhode, Y. Ma, J. Housden, R. Karim, C. A. Rinaldi, M. Cooklin, J. Gill, M. O'Neill, T. Schaeffter, J. Relan, M. Sermesant, H. Delingette, N. Ayache, M. W. Krueger, W. Schulze, G. Seemann, O. Dössel, and R. Razavi, "Clinical applications of image fusion

for electrophysiology procedures," in *Proc. ISBI 2012*, (Barcelona), pp. 1435–1438, 2012.

[152] S. A. Ben-Haim, D. Osadchy, I. Schuster, L. Gepstein, G. Hayam, and M. E. Josephson, "Nonfluoroscopic, in vivo navigation and mapping technology," *Nature Medicine*, vol. 2, pp. 1393–1395, 1996.

[153] L. Gepstein, G. Hayam, and S. A. Bemn-Haim, "A novel method for nonfluoroscopic catheter-based electroanatomical mapping of the heart," *Circulation*, vol. 95, pp. 1611–1622, 1997.

[154] P. A. Friedman, "Novel mapping techniques for cardiac electrophysiology," *Heart (British Cardiac Society)*, vol. 87, pp. 575–582, 2002.

[155] B. Pfeifer, F. Hanser, M. Seger, G. Fischer, R. Modre-Osprian, and B. Tilg, "Patient-specific volume conductor modeling for non-invasive imaging of cardiac electrophysiology," *The Open Medical Informatics Journal*, vol. 2, pp. 32–41, 2008.

[156] R. J. Schilling, N. S. Peters, and D. W. Davies, "Simultaneous endocardial mapping in the human left ventricle using a noncontact catheter," *Circulation*, vol. 98, pp. 887–898, 1998.

[157] C. C. Gornick, S. W. Adler, B. Pederson, J. Hauck, J. Budd, and J. Schweitzer, "Validation of a new noncontact catheter system for electroanatomic mapping of left ventricular endocardium," *Circulation*, vol. 1999, pp. 829–835, 1999.

[158] F. H. Wittkampf, E. F. Wever, R. Derksen, A. A. Wilde, H. Ramanna, R. N. Hauer, and E. O. Robles de Medina, "LocaLisa: new technique for real-time 3-dimensional localization of regular intracardiac electrodes," *Circulation*, vol. 99, pp. 1312–1317, 1999.

[159] M. W. Keller, S. Schuler, A. Luik, G. Seemann, C. Schilling, C. Schmitt, and O. Dössel, "Comparison of simulated and clinical intracardiac electrograms," in *35th Annual International Conference of the IEEE EMBS*, (Osaka, Japan, 3 - 7 July), pp. 6858–6861, IEEE, 2013.

[160] R. H. Milad El Haddad, "Algorithmic detection of the beginning and end of bipolar electrograms: Implications for novel methods to assess local activation time during atrial tachycardia," *Biomedi-*

cal *Signal Processing and Control*, 2012.

[161] S. Rusinkiewicz and M. Levoy, "Efficient Variants of the ICP Algorithm," in *Third International Conference on 3D Digital Imaging and Modeling (3DIM)*, 2001.

[162] K. S. Rhode, M. Sermesant, D. Brogan, S. Hegde, J. Hipwell, P. Lambiase, E. Rosenthal, C. Bucknall, S. A. Qureshi, J. S. Gill, R. Razavi, and D. L. G. Hill, "A system for real-time XMR guided cardiovascular intervention," *Medical Imaging, IEEE Transactions on*, vol. 24, pp. 1428–1440, 2005.

[163] B. R. Knowles, D. Caulfield, M. Cooklin, C. A. Rinaldi, J. Gill, J. Bostock, R. Razavi, T. Schaeffter, and K. S. Rhode, "3-D visualization of acute RF ablation lesions using MRI for the simultaneous determination of the patterns of necrosis and edema, journal=IEEE Transactions on Biomedical Engineering," vol. 57, pp. 1467–1475, 2010.

[164] H. M. Kjer and J. Wilm, "Evaluation of surface registration algorithms for PET motion correction," Studienarbeit, Technical University of Denmark, DTU, DK-2800 Kgs. Lyngby, Denmark, 2010.

[165] J. Wilm, "Iterative Closest Point," 2013.

[166] B. J. Scherlag, S. H. Lau, R. H. Helfant, W. D. Berkowitz, E. Stein, and A. N. Damato, "Catheter technique for recording His bundle activity in man," *Circulation*, vol. 39, pp. 13–18, 1969.

[167] G. K. Massing and T. N. James, "Anatomical configuration of the His bundle and bundle branches in the human heart," *Circulation*, vol. 53, pp. 609–621, 1976.

[168] H. Gray and W. H. Lewis, *Anatomy of the human body*. Philadelphia: Lea & Febiger, 1918.

[169] R. Schimpf, T. Reents, G. Hessling, I. Deisenhofer, A. Pflaumer, H. Estner, J. Wu, E. Ucer, B. Zrenner, T. Sueselbeck, J. Kuschyk, C. Veltmann, M. Borggrefe, and C. Wolpert, "[Magnetic navigation in invasive electrophysiological diagnostic and therapy]," *Herzschrittmachertherapie & Elektrophysiologie*, vol. 18, pp. 157–165, 2007.

[170] D. Potyagaylo, W. H. W. Schulze, and O. Dössel, "A new method for choosing the regularization parameter in the transmembrane potential based inverse problem of ECG," in *Computing in Cardiology*, (9-12 Sept. Krakow, Poland), pp. 29–32, 2012.

[171] R. Abächerli, R. Kobza, I. Christov, F. Frey, and P. Erne, "Do the ECG axis and intervals depend on the heart rate and on the body habitus?," in *Computing in Cardiology, 2011*, pp. 825–828, 2011.

[172] A. Henderson, J. Ahrens, and C. Law, *The ParaView Guide*. Kitware Clifton Park, NY, 2004.

[173] L. K. Cheng, J. M. Bodley, and A. J. Pullan, "Effects of experimental and modeling errors on electrocardiographic inverse formulations," *IEEE Trans Biomed Eng*, vol. 50, pp. 23–32, 2003.

[174] D. U. J. Keller, F. M. Weber, G. Seemann, and O. Dössel, "Ranking the influence of tissue conductivities on forward-calculated ECGs," *IEEE Transactions on Biomedical Engineering*, vol. 57, pp. 1568–1576, 2010.

[175] L. Wang, K. Wong, H. Zhang, H. Liu, and P. Shi, *Statistical Atlases and Computational Models of the Heart*, vol. 6364 of *Lecture Notes in Computer Science*, ch. How much geometrical detail do we need in cardiac electrophysiological imaging? a generic heart-torso representation for fast subject-specific customization, pp. 232–241. Springer Berlin / Heidelberg, 2010.

[176] F. M. Weber, D. U. J. Keller, S. Bauer, G. Seemann, C. Lorenz, and O. Dössel, "Predicting tissue conductivity influences on body surface potentials-an efficient approach based on principal component analysis," *IEEE Transactions on Biomedical Engineering*, vol. 58, pp. 265–273, 2011.

[177] R. Jones, W. H. W. Schulze, D. Potyagaylo, O. Dössel, and F. M. Weber, "Computing lead-field matrices for a body tissue conductivity range," in *Biomedizinische Technik / Biomedical Engineering*, vol. 58, 2013.

[178] R. Modre, M. Seger, G. Fischer, C. Hintermuller, D. Hayn, B. Pfeifer, F. Hanser, G. Schreier, and B. Tilg, "Cardiac anisotropy: is it negligible regarding noninvasive activation time imaging?," *IEEE*

Trans Biomed Eng, vol. 53, pp. 569–580, 2006.

[179] G. Seemann, D. U. J. Keller, D. L. Weiss, and O. Dössel, "Modeling Human Ventricular Geometry and Fiber Orientation Based on Diffusion Tensor MRI," in *Proc. Computers in Cardiology*, vol. 33, pp. 801–804, 2006.

[180] D. L. Weiss, D. U. J. Keller, G. Seemann, and O. Dössel, "The influence of fibre orientation, extracted from different segments of the human left ventricle, on the activation and repolarization sequence: a simulation study," *Europace*, vol. 9, pp. vi96–vi104, 2007.

[181] N. Toussaint, M. Sermesant, C. T. Stoeck, S. Kozerke, and P. G. Batchelor, "In vivo human 3D cardiac fibre architecture: reconstruction using curvilinear interpolation of diffusion tensor images," *Med Image Comput Comput Assist Interv (MICCAI)*, vol. 13, pp. 418–425, 2010.

[182] Y. Jiang, Y. Meng, D. Farina, and O. Dössel, "Effect of respiration on the solutions of forward and inverse electrocardiographic problems - a simulation study," in *Proc. Computers in Cardiology*, pp. 17–20, 2009.

[183] D. U. J. Keller, O. Jarrousse, T. Fritz, S. Ley, O. Dössel, and G. Seemann, "Impact of physiological ventricular deformation on the morphology of the T-wave: a hybrid, static-dynamic approach," *IEEE Trans Biomed Eng.*, vol. 58, pp. 2109–2119, 2011.

[184] Y. Jiang, D. Farina, and O. Dössel, "Effect of heart motion on the solutions of forward and inverse electrocardiographic problem - a simulation study," in *Proc. Computers in Cardiology*, pp. 365–368, 2008.

[185] M. Jiang, L. Xia, G. Shou, Q. Wei, F. Liu, and S. Crozier, "Effect of cardiac motion on solution of the electrocardiography inverse problem," *IEEE Transactions on Biomedical Engineering*, vol. 56, pp. 923–931, 2009.

[186] C. Han, S. M. Pogwizd, C. R. Killingsworth, and B. He, "Noninvasive reconstruction of the three-dimensional ventricular activation sequence during pacing and ventricular tachycardia in the canine

heart," *American Journal of Physiology. Heart and Circulatory Physiology*, vol. 302, pp. H244–52, 2012.

[187] H. P. Müller, P. Godde, K. Czerski, R. Agrawal, G. Feilcke, K. Reither, K. J. Wolf, and M. Oeff, "Localization of a ventricular tachycardia-focus with multichannel magnetocardiography and three-dimensional current density reconstruction," *J Med Eng Technol*, vol. 23, pp. 108–115, 1999.

[188] A. Thiagalingam, E. Wallace, A. Boyd, V. Eipper, C. Campbell, K. Byth, D. Ross, and P. Kovoor, "Noncontact mapping of the left ventricle: insights from validation with transmural contact mapping," *Pacing and Clinical Electrophysiology : PACE*, vol. 27, pp. 570–578, 2004.

[189] M. W. Krueger, W. H. W. Schulze, K. Rhode, R. Razavi, G. Seemann, and O. Dössel, "Towards personalized clinical in-silico modeling of atrial anatomy and electrophysiology," *Medical & Biological Engineering & Computing*, vol. 51, pp. 1251–1260, 2013.

[190] N. Smith, A. de Vecchi, M. McCormick, O. Camara, A. F. Frangi, H. Delin-gette, M. Sermesant, N. Ayache, M. W. Krueger, W. H. W. Schulze, R. Hose, I. Valverde, P. Beerbaum, C. Staicu, M. Siebes, J. Spaan, P. Hunter, J. Weese, H. Lehmann, D. Chapelle, and R. Rezavi, "euHeart: personalized and integrated cardiac care using patient-specific cardiovascular modelling," *Interface Focus*, vol. 1, pp. 349–364, 2011.

[191] D. Potyagaylo, W. H. W. Schulze, and O. Dössel, "Local regularization of endocardial and epicardial surfaces for better localization of ectopic beats in the inverse problem of ECG," in *Computing in Cardiology*, vol. 41, pp. 837–840, 2014.

[192] W. Schulze, D. Farina, Y. Jiang, and O. Dössel, "A Kalman filter with integrated Tikhonov-regularization to solve the inverse problem of electrocardiography," in *IFMBE Proceedings World Congress on Medical Physics and Biomedical Engineering*, vol. 25/2, pp. 821–824, 2009.

[193] W. H. W. Schulze, M. W. Krueger, K. Rhode, R. Razavi, and O. Dössel, "Non-invasive imaging of activation times in the atria - can

excitation patterns be reconstructed?," in *Biomedizinische Technik / Biomedical Engineering (Proc. BMT 2011)*, vol. 56, 2011.

[194] W. H. W. Schulze, M. W. Krueger, Y. Jiang, K. Rhode, F. M. Weber, D. Caulfield, B. R. Knowles, R. Razavi, and O. Dössel, "Localization of the Atrial Excitation Origin by Reconstruction of Time-Integrated Transmembrane Voltages," in *Biomedizinische Technik/Biomedical Engineering*, vol. 55, pp. 103–106, 2010.

[195] W. H. W. Schulze, D. Potyagaylo, H. F. Elies, and O. Dössel, "Training of a kalman filter with augmented measurement model on scar data for noninvasive cardiac imaging," in *Biomedizinische Technik / Biomedical Engineering*, vol. 57, p. 175, 2012.

[196] W. H. W. Schulze, D. Potyagaylo, and O. Dössel, "ECG Imaging - Workflow and Mathematical Concepts," in *Integrating Modalities and Scales in Life Science Imaging*, 2014.

[197] O. Dössel, M. W. Krueger, W. H. W. Schulze, F. M. Weber, and G. Seemann, "From atrial imaging and atrial mapping to atrial modelling," in *Cardiac Physiome Conference 2011*, (Merton College, Oxford), p. 58, Smith, N., 2011.

[198] O. Dössel, M. W. Krueger, F. M. Weber, C. Schilling, W. H. W. Schulze, and G. Seemann, "A framework for personalization of computational models of the human atria," in *Conf Proc IEEE Eng Med Biol Soc*, vol. 2011, pp. 4324–4328, 2011.

[199] D. Potyagaylo, W. H. W. Schulze, and O. Dössel, "Local regularization in the inverse problem of electrocardiography," in *Biomedizinische Technik. Biomedical Engineering*, vol. 58, 2013.

[200] D. Potyagaylo, E. G. Cortes, W. H. W. Schulze, and O. Dössel, "Synthesis and analysis models for sparse signal reconstruction in the inverse problem of ECG," in *Biomedizinische Technik / Biomedical Engineering*, vol. 59, pp. 941–944, 2014.

[201] A. Reinke, D. Potyagaylo, W. H. W. Schulze, and O. Dössel, "Geometrical model and corresponding conductivities for solving the inverse problem of ECG," in *Biomedizinische Technik / Biomedical Engineering*, vol. 59, pp. 937–940, 2014.

[202] D. T. Rudolph, W. H. W. Schulze, D. Potyagaylo, M. W. Krueger, and O. Dössel, "Reconstruction of atrial excitation conduction velocities and implementation into the inverse problem of electrocardiography," in *Biomedizinische Technik / Biomedical Engineering*, vol. 57, pp. 179–182, 2012.

[203] B. Wang, W. H. W. Schulze, and O. Dössel, "Non-invasive reconstruction of myocardial activation: a wavefront-based Tikhonov approach with tolerance operator," in *Biomedizinische Technik / Biomedical Engineering (Proc. BMT 2011)*, vol. 56, 2011.

List of Publications and Supervised Thesis

Journal Articles

- A. Loewe, W. H.W. Schulze, Y. Jiang, M. Wilhelms, A. Luik, G. Seemann, and O. Dössel, "ECG-based detection of early myocardial ischemia in a computational model: impact of additional electrodes, optimal placement and a new feature for ST deviation,", *BioMed Research International*, (accepted)
- W. H. W. Schulze, P. Mackens, D. Potyagaylo, K. Rhode, E. Tulumen, R. Schimpf, T. Papavassiliu, M. Borggrefe, and O. Dössel, "Automatic camera-based identification and 3-D reconstruction of electrode positions in electrocardiographic imaging," *Biomedizinische Technik. Biomedical Engineering*, 2014
- M. W. Krueger, W. H. W. Schulze, K. Rhode, R. Razavi, G. Seemann, and O. Dössel, "Towards personalized clinical in-silico modeling of atrial anatomy and electrophysiology," *Medical & Biological Engineering & Computing*, vol. 51, pp. 1251–1260, 2013
- D. Potyagaylo, E. G. Cortes, W. H. W. Schulze, and O. Dössel, "Binary optimization for source localization in the inverse problem of ECG," *Medical & Biological Engineering & Computing*, vol. 52, pp. 717–728, 2014
- N. Smith, A. de Vecchi, M. McCormick, O. Camara, A. F. Frangi, H. Delin-gette, M. Sermesant, N. Ayache, M. W. Krueger, W. H. W. Schulze, R. Hose, I. Valverde, P. Beerbaum, C. Staicu, M. Siebes, J. Spaan, P. Hunter, J. Weese, H. Lehmann, D. Chapelle, and R. Rezavi, "euHeart: personalized and integrated cardiac care using patient-

specific cardiovascular modelling," *Interface Focus*, vol. 1, pp. 349–364, 2011

Refereed Conference Articles

- W. H. W. Schulze, D. U. J. Keller, and O. Dössel, "A recursive cellular automaton that reconstructs transmembrane voltages with a range-adjusted Tikhonov-method," in *International Journal of Bioelectromagnetism*, vol. 13, pp. 184–189, 2011
- W. H. W. Schulze, F. Elies Henar, D. Potyagaylo, A. Loewe, M. Stenroos, and O. Dössel, "Kalman Filter with Augmented Measurement Model: an ECG Imaging Simulation Study," in *FIMH, LNCS 7945* (S. Ourselin, D. Rueckert, and N. Smith, eds.), pp. 200–207, Springer-Verlag Berlin Heidelberg, 2013
- O. Dössel, Y. Jiang, and W. H. W. Schulze, "Localization of the origin of premature beats using an integral method," in *International Journal of Bioelectromagnetism*, vol. 13, pp. 178–183, 2011
- D. Potyagaylo, M. Segel, W. H. W. Schulze, and O. Dössel, "Noninvasive Localization of Ectopic Foci: a New Optimization Approach for Simultaneous Reconstruction of Transmembrane Voltages and Epicardial Potentials," in *FIMH, LNCS 7945* (S. Ourselin, D. Rueckert, and N. Smith, eds.), pp. 166–173, Spinger-Verlag Berlin Heidelberg, 2013
- K. Rhode, Y. Ma, J. Housden, R. Karim, C. A. Rinaldi, M. Cooklin, J. Gill, M. O'Neill, T. Schaeffter, J. Relan, M. Sermesant, H. Delingette, N. Ayache, M. W. Krueger, W. Schulze, G. Seemann, O. Dössel, and R. Razavi, "Clinical applications of image fusion for electrophysiology procedures," in *Proc. ISBI 2012*, (Barcelona), pp. 1435–1438, 2012
- M. YingLiang, U. Mistry, A. Thorpe, R. J. Housden, Z. Chen, W. H. W. Schulze, C. A. Rinaldi, R. Razavi, and K. Rhode, "Automatic Electrode and CT/MR Image Co-localisation for Electrocardiographic Imaging," in *FIMH, LNCS 7945* (S. Ourselin, D. Rueckert, and N. Smith, eds.), pp. 268–275, Springer-Verlag berlin Heidelberg, 2013

Refereed Conference Abstracts

- W. H. W. Schulze, D. Potyagaylo, and O. Dössel, "Activation time imaging in the presence of myocardial ischemia: Choice of initial estimates for iterative solvers," in *Computing in Cardiology, 2011*, vol. 39, (9-12 Sept., Krakow), pp. 961–964, 2012
- A. Loewe, W. H. W. Schulze, Y. Jiang, M. Wilhelms, and O. Dössel, "Determination of optimal electrode positions of a wearable ECG monitoring system for detection of myocardial ischemia: a simulation study," in *Computing in Cardiology*, vol. 38, pp. 741–744, 2011
- D. Potyagaylo, W. H. W. Schulze, and O. Dössel, "A new method for choosing the regularization parameter in the transmembrane potential based inverse problem of ECG," in *Computing in Cardiology*, (9-12 Sept. Krakow, Poland), pp. 29–32, 2012
- D. Potyagaylo, W. H. W. Schulze, and O. Dössel, "Local regularization of endocardial and epicardial surfaces for better localization of ectopic beats in the inverse problem of ECG," in *Computing in Cardiology*, vol. 41, pp. 837–840, 2014

Conference Presentations

- W. Schulze, D. Farina, Y. Jiang, and O. Dössel, "A Kalman filter with integrated Tikhonov-regularization to solve the inverse problem of electrocardiography," in *IFMBE Proceedings World Congress on Medical Physics and Biomedical Engineering*, vol. 25/2, pp. 821–824, 2009
- W. H. W. Schulze, M. W. Krueger, K. Rhode, R. Razavi, and O. Dössel, "Non-invasive imaging of activation times in the atria - can excitation patterns be reconstructed?," in *Biomedizinische Technik / Biomedical Engineering (Proc. BMT 2011)*, vol. 56, 2011
- W. H. W. Schulze, M. W. Krueger, Y. Jiang, K. Rhode, F. M. Weber, D. Caulfield, B. R. Knowles, R. Razavi, and O. Dössel, "Localization of the Atrial Excitation Origin by Reconstruction of Time-Integrated Transmembrane Voltages," in *Biomedizinische Technik/Biomedical Engineering*, vol. 55, pp. 103–106, 2010

- W. H. W. Schulze, M. W. Krueger, K. Rhode, R. Razavi, and O. Dössel, "Critical times based activation time imaging," in *Proc. 38th International Congress on Electrocardiology*, 2011
- W. H. W. Schulze, D. Potyagaylo, H. F. Elies, and O. Dössel, "Training of a kalman filter with augmented measurement model on scar data for noninvasive cardiac imaging," in *Biomedizinische Technik / Biomedical Engineering*, vol. 57, p. 175, 2012
- W. H. W. Schulze, B. Wang, D. Potyagaylo, and O. Dössel, "Use of a tolerance operator in wavefront-based ECG imaging of transmembrane voltages," in *IFMBE Proceedings World Congress on Medical Physics and Biomedical Engineering*, vol. 39, 2012
- W. H. W. Schulze, R. Schimpf, T. Papavassiliu, D. Potyagaylo, E. Tulumen, B. Rudic, V. Liebe, C. Doesch, T. Konrad, C. Veltmann, M. Borggrefe, and O. Dössel, "Electrode arrangements for ECG imaging under practical constraints of a catheter lab setting," in *Biomedizinische Technik / Biomedical Engineering*, vol. 58, 2013
- W. H. W. Schulze, D. Potyagaylo, and O. Dössel, "Predicting the accuracy of cardiac pace mapping from lead field matrix characteristics," in *Proc. 40th International Congress on Electrocardiology*, 2013
- W. H. W. Schulze, D. Potyagaylo, and O. Dössel, "ECG Imaging - Workflow and Mathematical Concepts," in *Integrating Modalities and Scales in Life Science Imaging*, 2014
- W. H. W. Schulze, T. Fritz, D. Potyagaylo, J. Trächtler, R. Schimpf, T. Papavassiliu, E. Tülümen, B. Rudic, V. Liebe, C. Doesch, M. Borggrefe, and O. Dössel, "Effect of mesh resolution on forward calculations of the electrocardiogram in a simplified thorax model," in *Biomedizinische Technik / Biomedical Engineering*, vol. 59, pp. 945–948, 2014
- Z. Chen, J. Relan, W. Schulze, R. Karim, M. Sohal, A. Shetty, Y. L. Ma, N. Ayache, M. Sermesant, H. Delingette, J. Bostock, R. Razavi, K. Rhode, and A. Rinaldi, "Simultaneous non-contact mapping fused with CMR derived grey zone to explore the relationship with ventricular tachycardia substrate in ischaemic cardiomyopathy," in *Journal of Cardiovascular Magnetic Resonance*, vol. 15, p. P64, 2013

- O. Dössel, M. W. Krueger, W. H. W. Schulze, F. M. Weber, and G. Seemann, "From atrial imaging and atrial mapping to atrial modelling," in *Cardiac Physiome Conference 2011*, (Merton College, Oxford), p. 58, Smith, N., 2011
- O. Dössel, M. W. Krueger, F. M. Weber, C. Schilling, W. H. W. Schulze, and G. Seemann, "A framework for personalization of computational models of the human atria," in *Conf Proc IEEE Eng Med Biol Soc*, vol. 2011, pp. 4324–4328, 2011
- R. Jones, W. H. W. Schulze, D. Potyagaylo, O. Dössel, and F. M. Weber, "Computing lead-field matrices for a body tissue conductivity range," in *Biomedizinische Technik / Biomedical Engineering*, vol. 58, 2013
- D. Potyagaylo, W. H. W. Schulze, and O. Dössel, "Solving the transmembrane potential based inverse problem of ECG under physiological constraints on the solution range," in *Biomedizinische Technik / Biomedical Engineering*, vol. 57, p. 170, 2012
- D. Potyagaylo, W. H. W. Schulze, and O. Dössel, "Local regularization in the inverse problem of electrocardiography," in *Biomedizinische Technik. Biomedical Engineering*, vol. 58, 2013
- D. Potyagaylo, E. G. Cortes, W. H. W. Schulze, and O. Dössel, "Synthesis and analysis models for sparse signal reconstruction in the inverse problem of ECG," in *Biomedizinische Technik / Biomedical Engineering*, vol. 59, pp. 941–944, 2014
- A. Reinke, D. Potyagaylo, W. H. W. Schulze, and O. Dössel, "Geometrical model and corresponding conductivities for solving the inverse problem of ECG," in *Biomedizinische Technik / Biomedical Engineering*, vol. 59, pp. 937–940, 2014
- D. T. Rudolph, W. H. W. Schulze, D. Potyagaylo, M. W. Krueger, and O. Dössel, "Reconstruction of atrial excitation conduction velocities and implementation into the inverse problem of electrocardiography," in *Biomedizinische Technik / Biomedical Engineering*, vol. 57, pp. 179–182, 2012
- A. Thorpe, Z. Chen, W. H. W. Schulze, M. W. Krueger, J. Relan, H. Delin-gette, R. Razavi, C. Rinaldi, and K. Rhode, "Enhanced work-

flow for BSPM and ECGi using X-ray based Electrode Localisation," in *Bioengineering12*, 2012
- B. Wang, W. H. W. Schulze, and O. Dössel, "Non-invasive reconstruction of myocardial activation: a wavefront-based Tikhonov approach with tolerance operator," in *Biomedizinische Technik / Biomedical Engineering (Proc. BMT 2011)*, vol. 56, 2011

Supervised Student Theses

First Supervisor

- C. Ritter, *Imposition of Dynamic Model Based Regularization on the Solution in ECG Imaging*, Bachelor's thesis, Institute of Biomedical Engineering, Karlsruhe Institute of Technology (KIT), 2013
- E. R. Khaled Fattoh, *Solving the inverse problem of ECG for realistic atrial excitation propagation*, Student research project, Cairo University, 2013
- E. Mascareñas Marsal, *ECG Signal Processing for Inverse Electrocardiographic Imaging of Ventricular Extrasystoles*, Bachelor's thesis, La Salle, Universitat Ramón Llull, 2013
- R. Jones, *Towards a Personalized Volume Conductor Parameterization in ECG Imaging*, Bachelor's thesis, Institute of Biomedical Engineering, Karlsruhe Institute of Technology (KIT), 2013
- K. Vogel, *Wavefront-Preserving Regularization in Noninvasive Electrocardiographic Imaging of Ventricular Extrasystoles*, Student research project, Massachusetts Institute of Technology (MIT), 2012
- P. Mackens, *3D Reconstruction of ECG Electrode Positions from Multiple Photographic Images*, Bachelor's thesis, Institute of Biomedical Engineering, Karlsruhe Institute of Technology (KIT), 2012
- D.-T. Rudolph, *Non-Invasive Imaging of Cardiac Excitation Conduction Velocities*, Bachelor's thesis, Institute of Biomedical Engineering, Karlsruhe Institute of Technology (KIT), 2012
- B. Wang, *A Wavefront-Based Approach to Non-Invasive Reconstruction of Myocardial Activation*, Diploma thesis, Institute of Biomedical Engineering, Karlsruhe Institute of Technology (KIT), 2011

- F. Elies Henar, *Application of a Kalman Filter with Augmented Measurement Model in Non-Invasive Cardiac Imaging*, Master's thesis, Universitat Politècnica de Catalunya, 2011
- A. Loewe, *Comparison of Cardiac Simulation Tools Regarding the Modeling of Acute Ischemia*, Bachelor's thesis, Institute of Biomedical Engineering, Karlsruhe Institute of Technology (KIT), 2010

Second Supervisor

- Vynnie Kong, *ECG Imaging of Surface Transmembrane Voltages Using the Maximum A-Posteriori Method*, Student research project, Massachusetts Institute of Technology (MIT), 2014
- A. Reinke, *Regularization Parameter Estimation for the Inverse Problem of ECG*, Bachelor's thesis, Institute of Biomedical Engineering, Karlsruhe Institute of Technology (KIT), 2013
- E. Gil Cortés, *Spatio-Temporal Optimization Approaches to the Transmembrane Potential Based Inverse Problem of ECG*, Master's thesis, Universitat Politècnica de Catalunya / KIT, 2013
- M. Segel, *Improving ECG Imaging: Combined Regularization in Extracellular Space and the Space of Transmembrane Voltages*, Bachelor's thesis, Karlsruhe Institute of Technology (KIT), 2013

Awards & Grants

- Best Poster Award Computing in Cardiology 2012
- Young Investigator Award of the International Congress on Electrocardiology 2011

Supervised works:

- Best Poster Award Computing in Cardiology 2011 for Axel Loewe

Karlsruhe Transactions on Biomedical Engineering (ISSN 1864-5933)

Karlsruhe Institute of Technology / Institute of Biomedical Engineering (Ed.)

Die Bände sind unter www.ksp.kit.edu als PDF frei verfügbar oder als Druckausgabe bestellbar.

Band 2 Matthias Reumann
Computer assisted optimisation on non-pharmacological treatment of congestive heart failure and supraventricular arrhythmia. 2007
ISBN 978-3-86644-122-4

Band 3 Antoun Khawaja
Automatic ECG analysis using principal component analysis and wavelet transformation. 2007
ISBN 978-3-86644-132-3

Band 4 Dmytro Farina
Forward and inverse problems of electrocardiography: clinical investigations. 2008
ISBN 978-3-86644-219-1

Band 5 Jörn Thiele
Optische und mechanische Messungen von elektrophysiologischen Vorgängen im Myokardgewebe. 2008
ISBN 978-3-86644-240-5

Band 6 Raz Miri
Computer assisted optimization of cardiac resynchronization therapy. 2009
ISBN 978-3-86644-360-0

Band 7 Frank Kreuder
2D-3D-Registrierung mit Parameterentkopplung für die Patientenlagerung in der Strahlentherapie. 2009
ISBN 978-3-86644-376-1

Band 8 Daniel Unholtz
Optische Oberflächensignalmessung mit Mikrolinsen-Detektoren für die Kleintierbildgebung. 2009
ISBN 978-3-86644-423-2

Band 9 Yuan Jiang
Solving the inverse problem of electrocardiography in a realistic environment. 2010
ISBN 978-3-86644-486-7

Karlsruhe Transactions on Biomedical Engineering (ISSN 1864-5933)

Band 10 Sebastian Seitz
Magnetic Resonance Imaging on Patients with Implanted Cardiac Pacemakers. 2011
ISBN 978-3-86644-610-6

Band 11 Tobias Voigt
Quantitative MR Imaging of the Electric Properties and Local SAR based on Improved RF Transmit Field Mapping. 2011
ISBN 978-3-86644-598-7

Band 12 Frank Michael Weber
Personalizing Simulations of the Human Atria: Intracardiac Measurements, Tissue Conductivities, and Cellular Electrophysiology. 2011
ISBN 978-3-86644-646-5

Band 13 David Urs Josef Keller
Multiscale Modeling of the Ventricles: from Cellular Electrophysio-logy to Body Surface Electrocardiograms. 2011
ISBN 978-3-86644-714-1

Band 14 Oussama Jarrousse
Modified Mass-Spring System for Physically Based Deformation Modeling. 2012
ISBN 978-3-86644-742-4

Band 15 Julia Bohnert
Effects of Time-Varying Magnetic Fields in the Frequency Range 1 kHz to 100 kHz upon the Human Body: Numerical Studies and Stimulation Experiment. 2012
ISBN 978-3-86644-782-0

Band 16 Hanno Homann
SAR Prediction and SAR Management for Parallel Transmit MRI. 2012
ISBN 978-3-86644-800-1

Band 17 Christopher Schilling
Analysis of Atrial Electrograms. 2012
ISBN 978-3-86644-894-0

Band 18 Tobias Baas
ECG Based Analysis of the Ventricular Repolarisation in the Human Heart. 2012
ISBN 978-3-86644-882-7

Karlsruhe Transactions on Biomedical Engineering (ISSN 1864-5933)

Band 19 Martin Wolfgang Krüger
Personalized Multi-Scale Modeling of the Atria: Heterogeneities, Fiber Architecture, Hemodialysis and Ablation Therapy. 2012
ISBN 978-3-86644-948-0

Band 20 Mathias Wilhelms
Multiscale Modeling of Cardiac Electrophysiology: Adaptation to Atrial and Ventricular Rhythm Disorders and Pharmacological Treatment. 2013
ISBN 978-3-7315-0045-2

Band 21 Matthias Keller
Formation of Intracardiac Electrograms under Physiological and Pathological Conditions. 2014
ISBN 978-3-7315-0228-9

Band 22 Walther H. W. Schulze
ECG Imaging of Ventricular Activity in Clinical Applications. 2015
ISBN 978-3-7315-0374-3